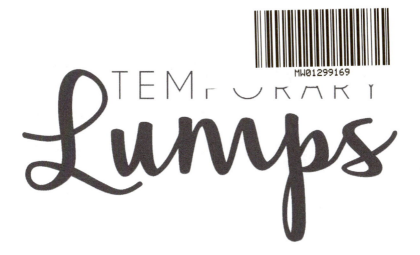

TEMPORARY Lumps

A journey of faith, perseverance and triumph#

Sonja B. Vaughan

Writer Book Publishing Services

*Melba—
Lumps are temporary...
Heaven is eternal!!
♡ Sonya*

Copyright © 2018 by Sonja Vaughan
All rights reserved

No part of this book may be reproduced or transmitted in any form or by any means without written permission of the author.

Published with Assistance from
Writer Book Publishing Services
www.writerbookpublishing.com

Printed and bound in the
United States of America

ISBN: 9781791379186

Temporary Lumps: A Journey of Faith Perseverance and Triumph
By Sonja B. Vaughan

DEDICATION

To my "Tribe"
For your unwavering love, prayers, support and comic relief

To Poom, Vera and Mrs. J
For being responsible for my love affair with words

WITH SPECIAL THANKS

To Andi Carlton
For the amazing front cover art. A picture is definitely worth a thousand words!

TABLE OF CONTENTS

Introduction	1
How We Got Here	4
This Is How We Do It!!	8
Pre-Game Prep	10
A Day of Gatherings	13
An Im-PORT-ant Day	16
Final Preparations	19
Day #1 is Done!	21
Making Progress	24
Figuring It All Out	27
In My Rearview Mirror	30
Yeah, It REALLY Happens!	34
Joy Bombs	38
Deep Couch Sitting	45
…A HAIRY Situation	49
Second Time Around	54
Just An Update	57
Community	60
Finding A Pattern	64
No More 3 x 5's	68
It Happens for a Reason	72
Pushing Through	77
You've Got Mail!	80
My Current Situation	85
Good Days and Bad Days	88
Treatment #3 In the Books!	91
I Knew it Had to Happen…	94
This Girl Is On FIRE	96
It Ain't All About Me	100

Positive People	104
Celebrate Good Times	109
Suck it up, Buttercup	112
Bits and Pieces	116
Vitamin Sea Therapy	119
Tackling Taxol	124
A Little Hiccup	128
Stinking Cold	132
No Bueno	136
Re-calculating	141
Giving Thanks	144
Rest is Best	147
Rounding Third and Heading Home	151
Just Plain Thankful	156
And We're Off...	161
Checking Them Off	164
Catching Up	167
Counting 'em Down	171
Is that a Finish Line in Sight?	176
Sooooo Close	181
Really Now?	185
And We're DONE!	189
Finding My New Normal	194
Thankful, Grateful, Blessed	199
A Few of my Favorite Things	202
Thinking Out Loud	207
Pneu-mo-WHAT?	210
Happy Spring, Y'all!	214
He is Risen!	218

INTRODUCTION

This is not your typical book. In 2017, I was diagnosed with breast cancer, and diagnosis in hand…..I decided to take to the internet and create a blog to keep friends and family in the loop. This book is a compilation of a year of my blog -- unedited and unrefined.

Although I love reading and writing, I am not a professional writer. What I am is one of over 250,000 women diagnosed annually with breast cancer. I started my journey full of unknowns and wrote about what I learned as it happened.

With cancer, God had presented me with a wonderful opportunity to share the good, the bad and the ugly of my chaos with friends and strangers who may be having similar struggles via the "interweb." Truly, in the midst of MY chaos, there became an awesome opportunity to share my faith, my fight and my story.

Sometimes, we find out that reality and our perception of reality are NOT the same. Life is going great……worries are few…..we're able to pay the bills…..everybody is healthy…..and we're feeling just fine about our station in life.

And then……without any warning, chaos ensues. For me, that "chaos" was a diagnosis of cancer. And somehow……purely by the grace of God……that chaos didn't break me.

It is my prayer that this compilation will help you through your cancer story, whether it's you or someone you love going through it. By putting my blog into a book form, it's my hope that you can take it with you wherever you go. You will likely be spending many hours in doctors' offices, and perhaps this blog-book can help you pass the time in a way that can lift your spirits.

At the very least, by reading my story, you will know you are not alone. Of course, you never were. I have never felt God's love more clearly than during my year of treatments. May you be encouraged, entertained and enlightened – completely at my expense! And oh – if you laugh a little along the way? Bonus!

Blessings!

Sonja

Esther 4:14 New International Version (NIV)
[14] *For if you remain silent at this time, relief and deliverance for the Jews will arise from another place, but you and your father's family will perish. And who knows but that you have come to your royal position for such a time as this?*

HOW WE GOT HERE
June 19, 2017

On April 18, 2017 - my life was pretty normal....well, there are those that would argue that I've NEVER been normal, but.....anyway, I had an appointment for my yearly OB/GYN visit. During that visit, I mentioned to my doctor that I had been experiencing some "tenderness" under my left armpit area. I really thought the underwire in my bra was causing it (probably due to a FEW extra pounds I'd put on) but felt it was worth mentioning.

After several attempts to locate the area of my "tenderness," the doctor found the culprit, a lump. My doctor was optimistic it was merely a cyst, due to the feel of it, and the fact that it was tender (everyone will tell you that cancer is not typically painful). He sent me for a mammogram and ultrasound to determine what it really was. I was able to get an appointment the same day. Mammogram appeared to show a cyst, while the ultrasound did not appear to show a cyst. The only way to know for sure was to do a biopsy. I was scheduled to come back in a week for a biopsy on April 26th, 2017. During the biopsy, the doctor saw yet ANOTHER mass that had not been apparent on either the mammogram or ultrasound the previous week. She biopsied BOTH spots.

The next 5 days were truly the LONGEST of my life.....waiting to hear the results from the biopsy. A phone call from the radiologist on May 1, 2107 confirmed that the biopsy results showed both spots tested positive for CANCER! Seriously? How can this be? How can I feel totally fine and healthy and have cancer? The pathology showed a Stage 2 Invasive Ductal Carcinoma - the mass measured 2.4 cm. I was blessed immensely and was able to see the surgeon that same week on Friday, May 5th. After consultation with her, I opted to have a lumpectomy + radiation in hopes of ridding myself of this beast. The lumpectomy was scheduled for Thursday, May 25th. Surgery went well, recovery was great. All that was left was to wait AGAIN for the pathology results that would let us know if we got clear margins.

A call from the PA on May 31st indicated that the doctor had NOT been able to get clear margins (the tumor was larger than it had appeared on the scans) and cancer cells were found in my Sentinel Lymph Node that was removed during surgery. The tumor was shaped a bit like a sea urchin - with tentacles going in many directions. Clear margins were achieved on 3 sides of the tumor.

Next we waited for radiation and medical oncology to review my pathology and recommend to the surgeon whether or not they needed to remove any additional lymph nodes when the re-excision surgery was done. Oncology recommended NOT removing any more lymph nodes - they would just target them with radiation. Surgery was set for June 8th, 2017. The surgery was successful and clear margins were obtained. Next up were visits with medical and radiation oncology at Duke University Cancer Center on June 14th. The long and short of it is that I will be needing 12 doses of chemo (4 doses of CEF or FEC - it's a combination of 3 drugs Cytoxan, Epirubicin and Fluorouracil) followed by 8 doses of Taxol. Once chemo is over, I may get a mini break and then start radiation. They have recommended 6 weeks of radiation at 5 days/week for a total of 30 doses of radiation. Doing a little bit of math in my head (which is NOT my strong point) it quickly became obvious that I would spend the majority of the rest of 2017 at Duke Cancer Center. While it's not the Ritz Carlton or as exciting as an all-inclusive vacation - I am oh so thankful that Duke Cancer Center is less than one hour from home. I am very fortunate to have such a world-class facility right in my back yard.

Thursday, June 15th CC and I spent over 1.5 hrs with the oncology pharmacist at Duke Cancer Center. She went over the first chemo regimen that I will be doing (CEF or FEC depending on your preference.....same drugs either way). She also spent a lot of time talking about the side effects and everything they do to try to minimize any nausea, sickness, etc. It was a very informative meeting. She sent me home with printed calendars with treatment days listed, when to take meds, what to do in event of fever - you name it, she prepared us for it. She said her goal was to make this treatment as boring as possible and hopefully to keep me as healthy as possible during this.

I am scheduled to have labs done and port put in on Monday, June 26, 2017 and I will start my first dose of CEF on Wednesday, June 28, 2017.

Pshew.....A LOT has happened since April 18th.

I have been journaling this mess since it started. Mostly because it was therapeutic and also because I wanted to be able look back on this and see all the ways that God blessed me in the midst of all of this "chaos that is cancer." I'm not a very private person - I probably "overshare"....but I truly felt like the more people that knew my story, the more people that I would have praying for me and the better off I would be. So this blog is my attempt at sharing my story. The highs and lows......the pretty and the not so pretty. If sharing my story encourages JUST ONE woman to get her yearly breast exam, then it will not be in vain......or if it encourages another breast cancer warrior who is fighting this same fight alongside of me, then I will count that as a blessing as well.

This much I know is true.......God's hands have been oh so apparent during EVERY. SINGLE. STEP. of this story so far. It's amazing just how many times HE has shown up and shown off and given me that not so gentle nudge letting me know that HE is right here with me and my family as we navigate the days ahead. I intend to give HIM all the glory for the big things and the small things.

Having a cancer diagnosis truly changes you in an instant. Your attitude.......your outlook.....your priorities......the ability to discern what things really matter and what truly is insignificant in the grand scheme of things.

So.....that's where we are right now. Here's to kicking this cancer right where it hurts! And the good news is - these were just "temporary lumps"....the real "lumps" have been removed from my body (Praise God) - but this cancer WILL NOT define me. This chaos that is cancer is just a "temporary lump" along the course of my life. I'm going to look back on this adventure one day and say "you know, it wasn't ALL bad."

I just met a new friend this weekend - she is a breast cancer survivor (just finished up her treatments around Thanksgiving 2016) and she said to me "the treatments were long and tough some days, but I was tougher!" I plan to look back on this mess and say the same thing.....that, with God's help, I was tougher than all the surgeries, doctors' appointments, lab work, scans, treatments, etc. Stay tuned to hear me make that same proclamation!

Disclaimer for those that don't know me personally, let me issue this disclaimer. I have a pretty warped sense of humor.....and have been known to make jokes about this cancer. It's not meant to be rude - it's just who I am. Laughing is much better than crying......and I'm choosing to laugh my way through this mess every chance I get!

Thanks for taking time to read my blog. I pray that you'll hang around with me for the rest of this ride and celebrate with me when we get to the finish line!

Blessings to you!

Sonja

THIS IS HOW WE DO IT!!
June 21, 2017

We planned our summer vacation months ago - and there was really no rhyme or reason to it other than my husband had 3 weeks available that he could take off. Two of those weeks would not work for us because Hunter would already be back in school in late August.....so our dates were chosen purely by the process of elimination! Clearly **"cancer"** wasn't in the picture when we picked our vacation.

Want to see how God works? The week that we had chosen months ago for our vacation turned out to be the week immediately BEFORE my chemo treatments are scheduled to start!! Amazing! Everybody hopes for sunny days when you are on vacation at the beach - and we are no exception. We've had some sunny days - but boy were they windy! We've managed to take the boat out one day so far - but between the wind and summer storms, the weather has not been in our favor to do the things we'd planned. Every time the guys get their fishing stuff together to walk out the door - down comes the rain again! The old Sonja would have been pissed......but "Cancer Sonja 2.0" (this is the title that Hunter gave me after my 2nd cancer surgery - that warped sense of humor runs deep at our house!) has kind of enjoyed the down time.....and just being here with my two favorite fellas. We've spent time on the deck watching the boats, shopping, watching TV, reading, playing Yahtzee and other games and oh yes - EATING!

It's quite possible I might have gained 10 pounds on this trip! I love food! All kinds of food - and while I know chemo affects everyone differently - many have said it changes their tastes. Things they loved no longer taste as good - and honestly, I've probably been more concerned over this stinking chemo messing with the tastes of my favorite foods than I have been over the chemo causing me to lose my hair. I mean, it's all about priorities, right???

Well, CC has given me free reign to eat any and everything I want this week. So guess what - I am trying hard not to disappoint him!!! So......this is how we do it....when things don't quite go the way WE had planned.......we EAT! CC is known for his "beach breakfasts." He's usually the first one up and he will get the griddle out and cook up a breakfast buffet. He never disappoints! We had breakfast with a view today.......eggs, pancakes, bacon, link sausage, toast, OJ...YUM! When we are in Morehead City, NC......El's Drive-In is a "must" stop EVERY. SINGLE. TIME. And don't forget Happy Cakes for the best cupcakes ever!

Even the best laid plans don't always work out......and often times, that's a good thing! We've not had the weather we hoped for - but we have had a lot of time together - eating, laughing, talking, fishing, and just enjoying each other. Clearly God knew ALL of us would need this time to rest, relax, refresh and recharge (oh, and REFUEL) before my chemo starts! Gotta run........somebody has to be in charge of planning that next meal! hahahaha!

Blessings!

Sonja

Psalm 116:7 New Century Version (NCV)#
7 I said to myself, "Relax, because the Lord takes care of you."

PRE-GAME PREP
June 24, 2017

We had a wonderful and relaxing vacation even if the weather wasn't in our favor every day. Now we are back home and taking care of business.

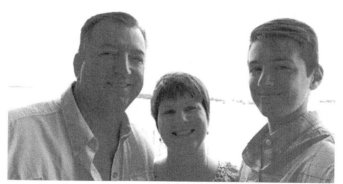
Living it up the week before chemo started

Today was "pre-game prep day!" Next week is a busy one.....Monday I have lab work done and my port placement followed by my first round of chemo on Wednesday. I spent some time today gathering lots of things I've been advised to have "on hand" for chemo.

While mom and I were at my oncology appointments last week, she brought her Scout bag and had some reading material, water, snacks, etc. in it. I love those bags - they are so lightweight and durable and I decided that's just what I needed to pack my chemo essentials in. Got me a Scout bag purchased and monogrammed (thanks Heidi)!

Here's some things I've been advised to have on hand:

- Everyone has said "take your iPad/computer to watch movies, or surf the net" so I made sure I got a bag large enough to accommodate my laptop.

- Candy to get the yucky taste out of my mouth when they flush my port.....Jolly Ranchers and Sour Patch candies were highly recommended (thanks Miranda) as well as orange Tic-Tacs!

- Hand sanitizer and baby wipes since infections are a no-no!

- Pedia-pops for days when I may not really want anything to eat.

- Migraine meds - since I suffer from migraines anyway, the pharmacist recommended I have them on hand for chemo day since we don't know how I will react to it!

- Biotene for dry mouth.

- Several different kinds of anti-nausea meds as well as a patch.

- Duke's Magic Mouthwash for mouth sores.

- Water......and more water......and more water......
- Snacks

- Lip balm to keep my lips moisturized

Pre-Game prep is done. Mission Accomplished! Hmmm........maybe I should have bought a larger bag! :-) I'm sure this list may grow - but I think I'm off to a good start! I'm sure I'll throw in a book also......even with all the e-books available on Kindle, I just like to hold a book in my hands. I bought a new book at the beach this week, but if anyone has any "must read" recommendations, let me know!

Happy Saturday everyone! Be awesome today and every day!

Hugs!

Sonja

Proverbs 21:31 New International Version (NIV)
[31] The horse is made ready for the day of battle, but victory rests with the Lord.

A DAY OF GATHERINGS
June 26, 2017

This day has been jam-packed! We started off attending 8:30am worship this morning. It was a day of celebrations! During the service, we commissioned 4 adults and 16 youth for an upcoming mission trip with ASP (Appalachian Service Project). Our group will be heading to rural Kentucky July 9th to do mission work there. This is the first time we've had youth old enough to attend ASP and we are all excited for them and the blessings they will both give and receive from this experience.

Next we celebrated our Youth Pastor, Curtis Hammock and his wife Dori. Curtis has recently been ordained as a licensed local pastor and today was his last day with us at Concord UMC! :-(While we are so happy that he has answered the call to serve as an ordained minister, we will surely miss him and Dori and their sweet children. It was truly bittersweet! Curtis and Dori - we love you guys and know that you and your family will be a blessing to your new congregation, just as you have blessed us over the past few years.

Sooooo many people took time to wish me well and offer encouragement for me this week as I embark on my chemo regimen. I continue to be amazed at the outpouring of love that has been showered on both me and my family through meals, calls, texts, cards, and visits. We have been oh so blessed by our church family, family, friends, neighbors and even strangers. Small town living ain't so bad - and from where I sit, it's times like this when folks truly show up and offer support in whatever form it is needed. I'm truly thankful for this community!

Church was followed by "Sunday Lunch at BJ's." My Aunt BJ prepared a table full of delicious food for lunch! I'm still amazed at how she manages to get so much food cooked in such a short window of time. I think she has some kind of super-power! I think everyone is trying to make sure I eat good to "beef up" for this chemo! :-) There has been no shortage of good food for me over the past few weeks! I completely forgot to get a picture of the meal she had prepared - sorry about that! But trust me when I say it was mmmm mmmm good!

Doctors' appointments and hectic schedules of late has kept me and the girls from being able to have our "therapy lunches." That stinks and we are going to rectify it soon! However - one of my therapy girls has had a full plate lately herself......so today I decided enough was enough - and that we needed an emergency therapy session! So we spent a few hours on the couch catching up and solving lots of problems. It was good for my soul!

The next thing you know, it's dinner time! Sunday dinners at my mom and dad's are always a treat! As I write this, I'm sure that you all must be thinking "Golly, she needs to be in a 12-step program for her food addiction!" Yeah - we love to eat around here. Mom had prepared a feast for dinner! So many of my favorites!!

And a wonderful blackberry cobbler compliments of Hunter Vaughan! Gran had a "training session" with him and Haden one day a few years ago and it was time well spent! These boys can cook!

Yes.....food and fellowship.....that's how we show love in this family. And trust me - there is an endless supply of that around here! Good times gathered round the table.....laughing, talking, debating......and arguing over who gets the last serving! :-)

What an awesome Sunday! So thankful for all the "gatherings" on this day. Every one of them was special.

Til next time!

Sonja

Romans 1:12 New International Version (NIV)
[12] *that is, that you and I may be mutually encouraged by each other's faith.*

AN IM-PORT-ANT DAY
June 26, 2017

Today got off to an early start. I left home around 7:30am to allow enough time to travel to Duke and get parked and make it to my 9:00 am lab appointment. They are so dang efficient in the Cancer Clinic Lab. You check in, get a pager (like the ones they give you at Outback when you're waiting for a table) and before you have a chance to get settled in your seat good, the pager is going off to let you know you're up next for labs! While I was standing in line to register, I got a message from my friend who just finished up her treatments about 6 months ago. She was wishing me luck and letting me know she was praying for me today! I just love those little "God-winks!"

Crazy how as many folks as they have back there doing labs, I got the same guy both times I've been. It was a sweet but short relationship, as I told him I was here today to have my port installed, so I guess that meant we would be officially breaking up. I told him it was truly nothing personal! :-) He took the news about the breakup better than I expected, and he wished me all the best going forward!

We had a little time to kill before my port appointment, so we ventured over to the Belk Boutique. My friend Miranda had told me that they had some items they gave to new cancer patients. I went in and asked about it, and sure enough there was a section of the boutique with scarves, hats, bandanas, toboggans, sleep caps, blankets, bracelets - lots of awesome items that were available to me. I chose a blanket (everyone says you will need it in the infusion room), a bandana and a awesome multicolored cap and a cool gift set! I opted to save a few of my freebies for later!

So I got a blanket, hat, bandana, moisturizer, Burt's Bees lip balm, toothpaste and hard candy from the Belk Boutique today!

Oh - and if you park in the parking deck and are there for labs, etc., you can get your parking ticket validated at the Belk Boutique also, and all day parking will only cost you $4.00. What a nice discount.

UPDATE My friend Barbara just advised me that you get FREE parking on chemo days. That's fantastic! Thanks for setting me straight Barbara!

A sweet friend took me to my appointments today. She is such a lovely person and has such a servant's heart. She asked the volunteer at the boutique if there were items they needed for the boutique to provide to cancer patients. The volunteer shared several ideas with her and I know she will share those ideas with our friends at church and provide them with some extra supplies in no time! We learned that the volunteer helping us was a 2 year breast cancer survivor and also a Christian. She shared some of her joys and struggles and the next thing I knew, my friend was joining us all in a circle and praying for her right there in the boutique! What a wonderful way to get our day started! God keeps showing up along this pathway!

Next up was my appointment for my port placement. My chemo doctor recommended the port be put in since I was going to have 12 chemo treatments. It makes it easier on the hospital staff and me also. I won't have to worry about bad, rolling or collapsed veins - they will be able to draw blood, deliver IV's, chemo, contrast, etc all through my port. The procedure was pretty painless - other than the lidocaine shot to numb my neck and chest. I'm a little sore around my neck and collarbone -

but that should not last too awful long. The stitches were internal and the incision is covered with surgical glue on the outside. I'm a little bruised - but nothing terrible. It feels a little weird having something like that implanted in my body - but they all assured me I would get accustomed to it being there.

So now I'm all geared up and ready for my first chemo treatment on Wednesday.

A friend sent this message today.....I loved it!

"One day down, is one day closer to the end!! "

It's all about perspective!

Keep the prayers coming ya'll!

Hugs!

Sonja

2 Corinthians 9:8 New International Version (NIV)
[8] *And God is able to bless you abundantly, so that in all things at all times, having all that you need, you will abound in every good work.*

FINAL PREPARATIONS
June 27, 2017

The "conscious sedation" meds they gave me yesterday wore off around bed time (wouldn't ya know). Whoever knew you used your neck/shoulder muscles so much when simply turning over in the bed!!! Goodness! And it just flat out feels weird having this port inside my chest! I'm bruised up a bit and it is a little tender to the touch - but the information they sent me home with yesterday says the soreness should wear off after 48-72 hours. I hope so! This, by far, has been more uncomfortable than the 2 lumpectomies! :-) Even so - I hate to complain. I'm thankful that I won't have to get "stuck" each and every time they need blood or give me chemo or IV meds.

I spent the day today tidying up lots of loose ends like paying bills and washing clothes. Then I went to see my hair girl Rachael. I realized last week that my next hair appointment was scheduled for tomorrow (June 28th) which was also the same day as my first chemo treatment. I called Rachael and told her to just cancel my appointment - especially since the medical oncologist had assured me that I would, indeed, lose my hair in the first 10-12 days after chemo. Rachael asked me to reconsider and to reschedule an appointment for today to go ahead and cut my hair shorter so when I start losing it, it wouldn't be such a drastic change!

I've worn my hair short before - it's been awhile (and SEVERAL pounds) ago - but I really like it! Talk about low maintenance! :-) It feels like puppy dog hair in the back! Thanks Rach..... <3

Several of you have asked me what I was going to choose to eat for dinner tonight - well......who is surprised that we had a Pizza Hut thin'n crispy Supreme Pizza AND a Pepperoni pizza. Good stuff right there!

I got my anti-nausea patch placed behind my ear around 7 pm per the pharmacist's directions.

Tomorrow will be a long day in the Cancer Center. My prayer is that I tolerate the chemo meds okay. I think I'm as mentally prepared as I can be. Thanks to all of you who have reached out to me today sending love and best wishes. Keep the prayers coming! Let's do this!

Be blessed!

Sonja

Matthew 6:34 New International Version (NIV)
[34] *Therefore do not worry about tomorrow, for tomorrow will worry about itself. Each day has enough trouble of its own.*

DAY #1 IS DONE!
June 28, 2017

Today was a busy day for the Vaughan household. We were up and out of the house by 8:15. CC had a return visit to Triangle Ortho regarding his herniated disc. He will go back on Monday for an injection to see if that provides any relief.

We left Triangle Ortho and headed to Duke Cancer Center. We had a little time to kill, so I perused the Belk Boutique and found some super cute hats and caps (Hunter helped me pick them out) and a nifty shirt that zips on each side to give easy access to your ports.

I had an 11 am appointment with my medical oncologists. Everything was good but they realized I had not had an echocardiogram as yet - and that is a MUST before starting chemo. They need your baseline readings, etc. Lucky for me - they were able to get me scheduled in the Cardiac Diagnostic Unit for 1:00 pm. I didn't actually get into a room until 1:30, but the technician worked really hard to get everything she needed to send to the cancer clinic to give them the go ahead to start treatment! They advised the infusion room that I was going to be a bit late, but I was still on the schedule to get my first dose TODAY!

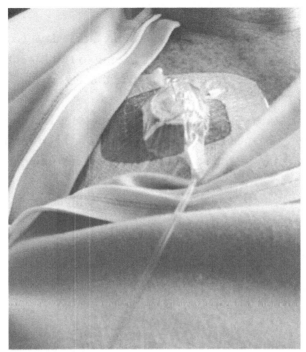

Thankful for my port and port-access shirt.

We were put back in the transfusion room a little after 3pm. I was given some zofran, decadron and ativan for anti-nausea first. Then they hung an IV of Emend for nausea as well. Next was a bag of Cytoxan, followed by 5 syringes of Epirubicin (it looked like red Jell-O)! And the final dose was the Fluorouracil which took about 5 minutes. After that, the only thing left to do was to put the Neulasta OnPro on my arm. This device will administer the Neulasta injection for me tomorrow night at the appropriate time. This thing is amazing. It pricked me shortly after she placed it on my arm.....and it somehow knows to wait from 24-27 hours and then start releasing the medication in my arm late tomorrow night. What a lifesaver - this little contraption saves me from having to go back to Duke every day after chemo to get a Neulasta shot. This OnPro is definitely the way to go!

Once the OnPro had been placed on my arm, we were all set to leave! I have to say, other than being tired, today was not that bad. No weird tastes in my mouth, no awful smells or allergic reactions to anything initially and I pray that continues.

I've been advised to rest as much as possible.....that days 1&2 are doable, but day 3 really has you feeling bad. I'm going to rest for sure - and I am praying that I won't feel super terrible over the next week.

Thanks to everyone who called, texted or messaged us today to check on me. That really means a lot. Again, we have been humbled by the outpouring of support for us during this time. You guys really are the best!

Blessings to each of you!

Sonja

Joshua 1:9 New International Version (NIV)
[9] *"Have I not commanded you? Be strong and courageous. Do not be afraid; do not be discouraged, for the Lord your God will be with you wherever you go."*

MAKING PROGRESS
July 1, 2017

My chemo went pretty smoothly on Wednesday, and I didn't have any severe side effects....Praise the Lord.

The oncology nurse placed a Neulasta OnPro on the back of my arm shortly after I had finished up with my chemo. Chemo puts everyone at a risk of infection. The Neulasta OnPro is an on-body injector that boosts your white blood cell count - thereby helping to reduce your risk of infection. Previously, you would have to go back to the hospital 23-27 hours AFTER chemo to receive a Neulasta shot. Now they have this nifty little device that attaches to either your arm or stomach. Once it's attached, it pricks your skin immediately and somehow this device knows when the appropriate amount of time has passed and then it beeps to alert you that it is about to start dispensing the medication in your arm. It takes about 45 minutes for the medication to be dispensed, and once it's done, the OnPro shows that it's empty and then you can remove it from your body. All of this happens wherever you are - without having to drive back to the clinic to get an injection. That was pretty dang cool! And I was very happy NOT to have to drive back to Duke at 6:00 pm at night just to get a shot!

I felt a bit queasy on Thursday and Friday even taking the anti-nausea meds. I'm not one to get up and eat right away, I need to be up a few hours before trying to put anything on my stomach. However, they have a pretty rigid schedule of times when I'm supposed to take these meds, and I think taking the meds plus eating when I wasn't really ready to eat just left me not feeling my best. I was pretty tired Thursday and Friday and just took it easy - laying around on the couch or enjoying some fresh air out on the screened porch. Everyone has advised me to "listen to my body" - and if it is telling me it needs to rest, then that's what I need to do. Sometimes that's easier said than done.

I've been really pleased with how I've tolerated the first round of chemo.....foods still taste the same to me, although I'm not wanting to eat an awful lot at a time. I've been experiencing dry mouth, so I am using Biotene toothpaste as well at Biotene mouthwash to help with that......and lots of hard candy.

The doctors said that the one thing that would buy me a trip to the hospital immediately would be dehydration. I've NEVER been a huge fan of water.....but I am doing my best to drink as much water or orange juice as I can. I prefer sleeping in my own bed!

Thank you all for your continued prayers and encouragement. I cannot tell you how instrumental those calls, texts, cards, food, milkshake deliveries, etc. have been in keeping my spirits up and just bringing a smile to my face. God has blessed me with so many prayer warriors and awesome friends supporting me in more ways than I ever could have imagined! I cannot fathom how folks fight something like cancer or any other illness without a network of friends and community of believers cheering them on. I am so thankful for my "village." It's pretty awesome when you don't even have to reach out to someone to ask for assistance - folks have been so good about seeing a need and just saying "I want to do this for you." It is quite an humbling experience - but I am thankful for each and every act of kindness that has been shown to my family and me since this whole mess started.

Hugs!

Sonja

1 Chronicles 16:11 New Life Version (NLV)
Look to the Lord and ask for His strength. Look to Him all the time.

FIGURING IT ALL OUT
July 4, 2017

Funny how things can be pretty dang awesome one minute, and all hell break loose the next. I was pleased with the way my body initially responded to the chemo last week. Wednesday through Saturday things seemed to be pretty normal. That all came to a screeching halt on Sunday. I felt good that morning and went to the early service at church. By the time lunch rolled around, I wasn't starving, but knew that I needed to eat something. I managed to eat a little bit of lunch, but wasn't feeling the greatest! I spent the rest of Sunday on the couch. Going to church and out to lunch did me in for the day! I was simply exhausted. Everyone tells me to "listen to my body" - so I was content to just hang out on the couch most of the day. I attempted to watch a movie with Hunter - but he advised me later that I fell asleep within the first 30 minutes of the movie!

Monday morning CC had to go to Durham for an Epidural Steroid Injection in an effort to get some relief for this pinched nerve in his neck. We have joked that we are just taking turns driving each other to doctor's appointments. I pray this injection gives him some relief. The tiredness continued most of the day on Monday - and even though I was being diligent about eating and drinking, nothing seemed to stay with me very long. Our neighbors cooked dinner for us - and everything tasted normal - but as had been the case all day, every time I got something on my stomach, it didn't stay there very long. ***I apologize for the TMI!*** I was plagued by diarrhea all dang day. Just when I thought I had been able to keep something on my stomach....well, it didn't happen. I got a bit nervous because I didn't want to get dehydrated. I definitely didn't want to end up in the ER for fluids. We read over my chemo instructions and the instructions there were to take Imodium to help with the diarrhea. I took one round of the Imodium last night and was able to get some relief and some sleep. That is.....until about 2:15 am. I woke up at 2:15 sweating like crazy. I got up and grabbed a thermometer to check my temperature. 100.5 is the magic number - I have been instructed to call my doctor and head to the ER if my temp reaches 100.5. My temperature was 100.0! I got me something to drink, took some Ibuprofen and stayed up awhile hoping to get my fever down. About an hour and a half later, my temp had dropped to 99 and I went back to bed.

There's a Community Wide breakfast provided every year on July 4th. Most of the time, we're at the beach and not able to attend.....but I wanted to go for a while today just to see friends and family that I don't get to see any other time. I had a few pieces of toast at home before we left and ate a little cantaloupe and watermelon. I had hoped to stay awhile and visit, but I was just so tired and weak we came home pretty quickly. I spent the majority of the day in the dark, cold basement. Rest is best! My fellas treated me to a banana milkshake this afternoon and that was quite yummy!

I know this, too, shall pass. Everybody tolerates chemo differently - and the effect it has on everyone's body is totally different. No two people's experience is the same. My main objective is to keep myself hydrated and fever-free and eliminate any trips to the ER!

Many have asked how to specifically pray for me - and right now, I would say to please pray for me to be able to stay hydrated and fever-free!

I have been so very blessed by the outpouring of love and kindness that so many have shown. I continue to be amazed at just how wonderfully God provides for his children - He knows our every need!

Happy July 4th!

Hugs!

Sonja

Philippians 4:19 New International Version (NIV)
[19] And my God will meet all your needs according to the riches of his glory in Christ Jesus.

IN MY REARVIEW MIRROR
July 6, 2017

What a difference a few days can make. Whether it's your life, your health, your outlook, or your attitude......having a chance to reflect on "what was" and "what will be" can truly be good for the soul.

Sunday through Tuesday of this week this cancer and chemo kicked my butt. BAM - outta nowhere, I was feeling fine and then.....not so much! I found myself disappointed that I wasn't feeling better, that I wasn't able to do something so simple as go to the grocery store by myself, that for a few days, cancer was "one-upping" me. But yesterday and today.....things shifted. I felt a bit better. And today - very clearly - I was able to see that even in those moments where I felt like crap, where my life was not like I would have wished it..........I was able to see that God was absolutely continuing to bless me even in the midst of all the ugly.

Last summer, our son Hunter spent over 30 days away from home. Between Scout Camp, a 2 week Out West Trip with his Scout Troop and a mission trip with his youth group - we saw our son very little. It was, indeed, a summer of growth for ALL of us. Yes, he's spoiled, but we have been very diligent about pushing him out of his comfort zone at times. He just needs a little push - and then he's fine. I firmly believe he's become a better kid because we've allowed him to venture away from us and experience life without us and on his own terms. Having a full summer last year, this summer we were all okay with scaling things back a bit. A week of summer vacation, a week of scout camp and a youth trip would be plenty. As luck would have it - his church youth trip and the week he would attend Scout Camp fell on the same dates - so he made the decision to attend Appalachian Service Project with his youth group. They will spent a week in rural Kentucky doing mission work and helping do service projects like build porches, paint houses, etc. (they leave this coming Sunday)!

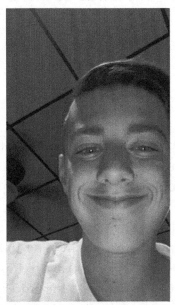

This kid right here......ya'll, he's been such a blessing his entire life, but especially the past few weeks!

I realized yesterday just how much I'm going to miss this kid next week while he's away - for reasons totally different than in the past. This fella has been my constant companion and sidekick since school was out. He has been stuck at home this summer with a mom with cancer and dad out of work on disability due to a herniated disc. He's had to pick up some slack and he's done it with a Servant's Heart! He's not let me overextend myself. He's always saying, "mom, I can do that, you don't need to!" He's always made me proud - but I've been extremely proud of the "can do" attitude he has maintained over the past few months. He grocery shopped for last night's dinner - and he prepared and cooked it by himself. Dad drove him to the grocery store, but he took my list and came back with everything we needed to prepare our delicious meal! I lit the grill for him and dad supervised - but otherwise, he was in charge. Not sure who was more proud!

So looking in my rearview, while I felt badly that his summer would not be as adventurous as last......turns out God knew we were going to need him here with us this summer. I know it wasn't the summer he had planned either - but we are all going to make the best of it! I've promised him a fun "reward/make-up" vacation when this "shit storm" is over. I intend to make good on that promise.

And then there's his dad. Our workaholic provider - always, always working to make sure we have everything we need and then some. CC has been out of work unexpectedly since early June when he was diagnosed with a herniated disc/pinched nerve. He has been in excruciating pain up until this past Monday, when he was FINALLY able to get an epidural steroid injection and some relief of the constant pain. While it's never fun to have two sick folks in one household at the same time - there have been some blessings of both of us being "out of commission" at once. We've joked that we have taken turns taking each other to doctor's appointments. Thankfully our "bad" days have not come at the same time! He and Hunter were both able to accompany me to my first chemo treatment. That was good for me - to have them there, to see that it wasn't awful, to know what goes on. Under normal circumstances, he would have had to take vacation time to accompany me, or work a Saturday to make up for the day off during the week.

Coincidence? I think NOT! It's nothing but "God-incidence" that our summer has turned out exactly like it has. God's timing and God providing. Providing caregivers for me when I didn't know I would need them. Providing a cheering section for me on the days I feel like crap.

So you see......looking through the rearview mirror TODAY - it turns out my Sun-Wed was not really all that bad. It stunk a little bit at the time - but I can look back now and see how that even in the midst of all that ugly - God was continuing to bless me and provide for me. Allowing me to have two wonderful caregivers right within arm's reach.

We continue to reap unexpected blessings each and every day. Phone calls to say "I'm bringing food," folks just showing up with food, folks providing meals and texting notes of encouragement from all corners of the world, emails to say "I'm going to do this for you"......we have been so very blessed!

Today I'm thankful for my rearview mirror. Thankful that life looks much clearer through my rearview, and thankful that my windshield gives me a much bigger view of where I'm actually heading!

Blessings!

Sonja

Proverbs 4:25 (NIV)
[25] *Let your eyes look straight ahead; fix your gaze directly before you.*

YEAH, IT REALLY HAPPENS!
July 9, 2017

Consider yourself warned!!! This post will be a bit different than my previous posts. Sure, there'll be some bad humor - that's a given. But you see, the deal I made with myself when I decided to journal this "chaos that is cancer" was that I wanted to be as real, open and honest and authentic about this **"lump in the road"** as I could (sorry ya'll, I just CANNOT bring myself to refer this as a **"JOURNEY"** - it just sounds so cliché'). My goal was to share the good, the bad and the ugly......and all the in between.

While none of us just sit around and try to borrow trouble - I'm sure that MOST of us - at some point - have looked around at folks in our church, community, family, etc and witnessed them going through a difficult time - we may have thought to ourselves "if I were ever to have _____(enter your chosen diagnosis here), I know that as awful as it would be, I would ALWAYS be able to count on _____(enter the name(s) of folks in your circle of influence here) to be there for me.

Stop and think for a minute of the names of folks you would use to fill in that blank. Family, friends, church family, neighbors, coworkers, PTA friends, Jr. League friends, your oldest and dearest friend from elementary school........the list goes on and on. You get the picture, right? We all have our mental "go-to" list of folks that we are CONFIDENT will be there for us in both good and bad times.

Well.....I hate to burst your bubble......but you can most certainly expect that there will be one or two folks on your "go-to" list that will surprise (or disappoint) you. They won't show up. They won't call. They won't text. They won't send flowers or food. They won't be there in your cheering section like you had imagined. And you will just not be able to wrap your chemo brain around it! The reasons for this are many. Here's just a quick list of a few reasons some friends and I have come up with.....

CANCER scares the hell out of some people - maybe they lost a loved one to a similar diagnosis, it may bring up painful memories of prior loss, etc

- some people just truly DO NOT know what to say

- some people don't deal well with "less than perfection" (sad but true) they can't handle a "sick" friend coming over to dinner with their "normal" friends

- some people don't handle the physical changes that occur as a result of your illness

- some folks just don't want to deal with your illness - it's an inconvenience to them

I could go on and on, but I think you get my drift.

My Aunt BJ told me years ago that "not everybody or every family knows how to deal with sickness." I wasn't exactly sure what she meant at first. But we talked about how our family had seen its share of illnesses......from heart disease, to lung cancer, breast cancer, colon cancer, a paralyzed family member, strokes and several other illnesses. As unfortunate as it was, our family has been forced to play the hand that we have been dealt. In our family - we learned to "deal with sickness." Hospitals, waiting rooms....receiving good news and not-so good news. Many families never have to experience a lot of sickness and as a result, often don't know how to deal with sickness of others when the time comes. **#truth**

I've been reading a book called "CANCER Now What?" by Kenneth C. Haugk, Ph.D. It's a great read. This book is excellent whether you are the one diagnosed with cancer or if you are a family member or caregiver to someone with cancer. It's more like a "how-to" book regarding cancer and you can read it front to back or skip around to specific sections that may be relevant to you at the present time. I'd been pondering writing about these relationship changes but wasn't sure if I'd offend folks or not - but after praying about it and then seeing it referenced in Dr. Haugk's book, I felt like that was my sign that this was, indeed, a "real" issue and I felt the need to share it. Dr. Haugk says "Some relationships may grow more distant," but, "you may also develop new, close relationships." And for those who do at first distance themselves from you, "the change isn't necessarily permanent." Dr. Haugk also points out that while some relationships won't change at all, some can change in a way that "may be disappointing." I recommend you buy and read Dr. Haugk's book – it helps you mentally prepare for changes. However – I have a few thoughts that might be helpful to you, too!

Don't despair!! This post isn't going to end on a bad note! I can personally attest to the fact that I have seen first hand how a few of those on my "go-to" team did not show up. Disappointing.......of course. But trust me - when you "catch the cancer" like I have, things that would have wrecked "pre-cancer Sonja" fall like water off a duck's back from "Cancer Sonja 2.0." Your outlook and perspective COMPLETELY change! And I promise you that for each person on your "go-to" team that does not show up........you can rest assured that there will be AT LEAST one person (but probably more) that you may never have known before that will take the place of those you had imagined! It may be a brand new friend/survivor you meet in a chance elevator encounter who you bonded with immediately and has continued to keep up with you via text messages.......or it may be a friend of a friend of Aunt So-and-So's that heard your story and felt compelled to bring food and visit......just because........or someone at church........or someone you meet at chemo....... You see what I'm saying, right? While it may seem devastating or disappointing at first - you will quickly move on.....and realize that God has already arranged for the right folks to be in your path......no matter how you know them or don't know them. God has sent so many "unexpected" people my way in the first few months of my diagnosis. It continues to amaze me - but I promise you God sends us who and what we need.......at just the right time.......every time!

Now for a quick update on me. I have felt like a new person since Friday. Food has been staying with me.......I've had some decent energy. Still can not stand up on my feet for long periods of time without feeling totally wiped out. Awful indigestion (and I've learned indulging in watermelon is no help for that). I get very hot and sweaty and nervous. I'm sleeping okay. My port is still causing me some sleeping issues - but hopefully that will all work itself out in time. I'm praying for a great week!

I will be minus my sidekick this week. He left at 6:00 am this morning headed to Kentucky to do mission work with his youth group for Appalachian Service Project. I will surely miss him but know he will have a great experience and have LOTS to tell me when he gets home! Praying they have a wonderful week and shine for Jesus! Tomorrow I have an adventure planned. More to come on that. Wish me luck! Until then.....

Sonja

Isaiah 49:23 New International Version (NIV)

[23] *"Kings will be your foster fathers, and their queens your nursing mothers. They will bow down before you with their faces to the ground; they will lick the dust at your feet. Then you will know that I am the Lord; those who hope in me will not be disappointed."*

JOY BOMBS
July 11, 2017

In Margaret Feinberg's Bible Study "Fight Back With Joy" - the participants were asked to write down 3 "joy bombs" everyday. **"Joy-bombs"** are defined as things that bring us joy (big or small). And things that.....when they happen.....you just KNOW it was God! I admit I have not done the Bible Study - I hope to someday soon - but I have read the book "Fight Back With Joy" that the study was based on (which was gifted me to shortly after my diagnosis from a sweet friend).

I simply CANNOT say enough good things about this book. First of all, Margaret and I could be sisters from another mister. Our personalities seem to be a lot alike! I loved her spunk and her grit - and her refusal to let cancer steal her joy! If you know someone who has been diagnosed with cancer and want to do something for them......gift them this book and take them a milkshake! They will thank you!

Anyway......I received the text below on Sunday from a forever friend.....she's been around as long as I have been alive! :-) We joke and kid a lot - but we can be serious every now and then. Here's the text she sent me:

> Sunday 7:56 PM
>
> You looked great today. Any trips to duke this week. I'm praying for you to have a wonderful week with many "joy bombs" coming your way. Learned that word in a recent Bible study when you just look up and say thank you Lord I know you did that
>
> Love you.

So we texted back and forth awhile and I smiled at her reference to "joy-bombs."

JOY-BOMB#1
FINDING THE RIGHT ONE!

Monday, I had a big "joy-bomb" - I had a friend offer to take me shopping for my "cranial prosthesis." Google it. It is a thing. I wasn't feeling 100% but I felt like I just needed to push through and let God take care of the rest. We had an amazing trip! We had the best time chatting on the ride to and from Raleigh and my shopping experience was fantastic. Like, it's a real problem when you have a difficult time deciding WHICH cranial prosthesis you want to buy! I didn't really think I'd want one - I'm more a baseball cap kinda girl......but my friend Dianne (who is a 2x breast cancer survivor) had a long talk with me a few weeks ago and asked me to reconsider. She said there would be many days that I felt like crap and could care less how I looked.......BUT.....she also said that there would be some really good days when I felt spunky and felt like going out and having fun and looking my best - and on THOSE days, there might be an occasion or an event that I would want to attend and I would WANT to look my best and quite simply - there were some things that a baseball cap just wasn't appropriate attire for! As I left her condo that day - she said to me firmly "GET THE WIG!"!! So Dianne.......I actually listened to you and took your advice!

Don't be jealous! And Shelly M - sorry to disappoint. No Katy Perry purple!

Clearly Joy-Bomb#1 was a successful shopping trip for my cranial prosthesis! I just love saying that!

JOY-BOMB #2
FROM A FRIEND SINCE JUNIOR HIGH

So today......not feeling the worst, and not the best, but off to a slow start. Finally showered and headed to the pharmacy to pick up some meds. Literally while standing at the counter waiting on my meds, this message popped up on my phone.

> 1:14 PM
>
> Thinking about you and sending you good vibes and prayers for strength today!!
>
> Just heard Mercy Me's Even If and YOU popped in my head 😊
>
> >> You are soooo sweet! I love getting "joy bombs" like this!!
>
> It's funny how the Holy Spirit just lays someone right on your heart out of the clear blue sky 💜 Hope your day is just perfect 😊

JOY-BOMB #3

Less than an hour later, I saw a sweet friend who spent some time with me catching up and gave me a sweet card about our friendship......and 2 thoughtful gifts! Joy-Bomb#3 for the day! Holy cow! Literally - all of these things occurred out of the blue - unexpectedly - and each a wonderful blessing from both the Lord and the giver.

JOY-BOMB #4

Later tonight, I'm checking Instagram hoping maybe one of our youth has posted some pics of their trip (yeah, cause it's awfully quiet around here without Hunter). Well, I didn't find any pics but I did find a message sent to me from another friend that I had not heard from in years until just a week or so ago. Literally.

> Hey Sonja- I'm checking on you to see how you're doing and feeling. You're in my prayers.

Are ya'll hearing and seeing this? My wild and crazy friend on Sunday told me she was praying for a week filled with Joy-Bombs. Can I say it's only Tuesday and I can hardly wait for the rest of the week??? Can you see how God is working in all of this. My friend prayed for this........and God answered.......in ways unexpected and unimagined! Many have been praying for me and my family - and He is definitely hearing and answering those prayers.

The very idea that my name was put on someone one's heart to think about me is so humbling......but then for them to ACT on that and in turn let me know that I crossed their mind brings so much comfort and joy to me. I love how God keeps letting me know that He is right on top of this and He is in this with me and He will NEVER EVER leave me nor forsake me! I know we've all had someone cross our minds in what may seem like a totally weird and crazy time. I'm learning to take those times to reach out to the person just to say - you were on my mind. I believe God has them cross our minds for a reason!

Does having cancer suck? Why, yes, indeed it does! But I would be lying if I didn't say that since being diagnosed with cancer, I have seen and felt the amazing love of God more than I have at any time in my life. I have had people love on me and my family in ways I never imagined. I have felt His peace that passes all understanding literally from Day 1. I'd always heard about that peace - but I truthfully never really understood it until I FELT it myself. Do you have to have cancer to receive joy-bombs? Absolutely not! WE JUST HAVE TO LOOK FOR THEM!

I think when life is good and things are going great - we all get so busy that we don't take time to truly appreciate the small stuff. It gets all buried in the minutia of the day. Does having cancer give me a keener eye for joy-bombs? No doubt!! And you know what - even after the good Lord and these doctors evict this cancer from my body......I pray that I will maintain that keen eye for joy-bombs!

And literally since I've been working on this blog post, I've received several other "joy-bombs." I'd never wrap up this post if I detailed them all. And ya'll, I've had so many people send me joy-bombs - please, please, don't feel like your act of kindness was any less important if I didn't highlight it here! That's so not what this is about! These were just some quick and easy ones for me to use!

I was a little leery when starting this blog. You never know how something like this will be received. But in the short time I've been doing it, I have been encouraged by many of you taking time to send notes, comments, etc. Just today, in a conversation with someone about my blog - I shared my reasoning for doing this......

> *It's therapy for me....and it's selfish too in that I'm sure months from now some of this will be difficult to remember. I wanted a way to document the whole ordeal. Good and bad and be able to look back and see just how far I came and hopefully how it really*

wasn't as bad as you imagine and most importantly to document the places God shoes up....in the midst of this....and just seeing how many people we have praying for all of us.....and how in crazy weird ways this may help somebody else....or force someone to get a mammogram....or send a card or text to someone when they cross their minds. I know God didn't give me cancer. I didn't want it but your kid didn't ask for asthma either. We do the best we can with what we are given. I would like to think that if this cancer and this blog gives me a platform to encourage just a few then it will be worth it! I refuse to let this cancer be in vain. I need to make it count for something!! And sweet folks like you encouraging me are an added bonus!!!

So here's the crazy thing. Many don't know that my degree is in English with a concentration in Communications/Public Relations. It's been a running joke I have never really had a job that "utilized" my degree to the full extent. Yeah - don't go calling the grammar police - I know this blog is not grammatically correct and I kinda like it that way.

But I'd be lying if I hadn't thought about the fact that here......at 50 years of age.....sooo many years after obtaining my degree......isn't it kinda crazy to think that maybe this had been my purpose all along?

That having cancer would give me the kick in the butt that I needed to just put myself out there and use that degree for something to make me feel better about my situation......and hopefully help or inspire a few folks......and be able to give God all the glory for it?

Call me a late bloomer if you will - but I'll take it! We need to bloom where we are planted, right?

Blessings......and praying that each of you take the time to stop and look for your "joy-bombs" each day!

I'd love to hear from you when you receive them! :-)

Hugs!

Sonja

Psalm 139:16 The Message (MSG)

¹³⁻¹⁶ Oh yes, you shaped me first inside, then out; you formed me in my mother's womb. I thank you, High God—you're breathtaking! Body and soul, I am marvelously made! I worship in adoration—what a creation! You know me inside and out, you know every bone in my body; you know exactly how I was made, bit by bit, how I was sculpted from nothing into something. Like an open book, you watched me grow from conception to birth; all the stages of my life were spread out before you, The days of my life all prepared before I'd even lived one day.

DEEP COUCH SITTING
July 7, 2017

Most of you have seen the Swiffer commercial with Big Jerry - the dad who has a rambunctious son that doesn't allow him much time to sit down and do any "deep couch sitting!" I like that term "deep couch sitting!" It always made me chuckle.

Well.....let me tell ya......the past two days, I have done some "deep couch sitting." Tuesday night, I wrote out a list of 5-6 things I wanted to accomplish on Wednesday. Nothing major - send some emails, write some checks, a few menial tasks that surely I could cross off my list by lunch time the next day.

Yeah......not so much!

As soon as I got out of bed, my stomach was giving me a fit. Not the way you want to crawl out of bed already feeling yucky. I walked to the kitchen, made some coffee and plopped down on the couch. Hoping if I somehow "eased" my way into Wednesday, my tummy would come around. Three trips to the bathroom by 10:30 am is not ideal when you didn't get up until 8:00ish. Imodium is my new best friend......this week. I hope it's a short-lived friendship! Other than taking a shower - I spent ALL DAY Tuesday on the couch. I was doing some "deep couch sitting" and "deep couch lounging!" And you know what - I am COMPLETELY okay with that. ZERO of my items got checked off my "to do" list......so I simply rolled them over to Thursday! I'm learning to give myself some slack if I can't do all the things I think I should be able to.

I continue to be amazed how you can feel great one minute and BAM - the next minute you feel like something has sucked every ounce of energy out of you. I'm trying to keep a record of how I feel each day. I want to see if there is a "pattern." Like will chemo days 1-4 be normal and I will feel fine......and will days 5-9 be days with lots of nausea and diarrhea and will things get better after day 10. We'll see. Maybe.....maybe not. It's worth checking out anyway.

Today was better. I got those items checked off my list. Mom took me to town to pay some bills and run a few errands. It seems that 3-4 hours is about the maximum amount time I can be out and about before I crash and head to the comforts of my couch. "Listen to your body" is what everyone says. I'm really trying to do that. I rested most of the afternoon and felt good enough to have a "date night" and have dinner out with friends. It was a great time. Much needed time with friends - and lots of laughter.......which truly is good for the soul.

So you guys know that I knew NOTHING of blogging before starting this blog - and I really don't know much more now about all the intricacies of blogging. I've been fooling around with the owner dashboard section a little bit trying to figure out all the intricacies of this blogging thing. Well, there is this neat STATS section where it shows you how many people have viewed your page each day, etc. And then there's this map of the world and it highlights the places that my blog has been read. I was completely and utterly amazed to realize all the places that my blog had been read!!!

- United States

- United Kingdom

- Turks & Caicos Islands

- United Arab Emirates

- Russia

- India

- Aruba

- Canada

What??? Seriously?? This whole internet and social media thing continues to amaze me!

So yesterday morning, I get a message from a former co-worker that I haven't seen in years. She told me that her mom had been diagnosed with breast cancer shortly after me and she told me that her mom had been reading my blog and how it had been a blessing for them. Now.....my friend lives in NYC.....and her mom lives in Tennessee. I think that's when it really hit me that folks outside of our little community were actually reading my blog! I never......ever imagined such would be the case! And ya'll, I just have to tell you how God worked in my friends life. Her mom got diagnosed with cancer in Tennessee. My friend is in NYC. Three days later.....do you hear me.....THREE DAYS LATER.....my friend got laid off from her job in NYC with 6 months severance. Now - under normal circumstances, I know the layoff would have been devastating. But you see - this layoff allowed her to simply pack her bags and head home to Tennessee to be a caregiver for her mom! God truly works in mysterious ways! Her mom had her first treatment today....and she was able to be right by her side! :-) If that isn't God smiling on ya, I don't know what is!

I also get a text from another friend yesterday telling me that a 33 y/o coworker had been diagnosed with breast cancer and would be starting treatment soon. If that wasn't bad enough - this young lady is 17 weeks pregnant. I. SIMPLY. CANNOT. IMAGINE. Suddenly.....my cancer chaos did not seem like such a big deal. My heart was so heavy for this young lady and what she must be going through physically, mentally and spiritually. I just wished I could squeeze her really, really tight and tell her that she is stronger than she can possibly imagine and that she can do this.......and to never, ever, give up and that she is NOT alone!

Cancer does not discriminate. It doesn't matter your age, your race, your socio-economic standing, your education, your political affiliation, your sex......it is no respecter of persons. Cancer Sucks......PERIOD!

I'm thankful for a day of "deep couch sitting." However, I advised my husband that I'm pretty sure, when this is over - we may definitely need to invest in a new couch - I'm pretty sure I'm wearing some permanent "holes" in this one!

Blessings,

Sonja

Psalm 29:11 The Message (MSG)
[11] God makes his people strong. God gives his people peace.

...A HAIRY SITUATION
July 16, 2017

I've had an uneventful few days.......feeling good, but tire quickly. I've OD'd on Food Network TV and Hallmark Movies (much to my hubby's dismay) and done some reading. Not a bad few days. And best of all - I got my sidekick back late Saturday afternoon! All is good in my world!

The day I first met my medical oncologist and she recommended my chemo regimens to me, she looked at me and, quietly..... but matter-of-factly said...... "you WILL lose your hair."

I asked her if she knew how soon that would happen and she said typically within 10-12 days.

My first treatment was on June 28th......and it was only this past Wednesday (July 12th) that I noticed my hair showing up on the bathroom counter after I towel dried my hair. I made it 14 days before it was noticeable. She was pretty on-target!

The bathroom counter was covered in hair this morning and CC gathered a large glob out of the shower

Yeah - this is really happening! Since Hunter was away all week at ASP, my prayer was that it would not all come out before he got home. I didn't want him coming home to a bald mom!

I thought that might be a bit traumatic even for him! It was noticeably thinner than before he left and in true Hunter fashion - he noticed right away!

He likes to tap me on my head anyway - and when he did, I cautioned him "be careful, it's falling out like crazy!"

Of course, he didn't believe me - but he asked me if he could try to "pull" a piece out I said sure! I don't think he was prepared for how easy it was going to come out!

He was like "oh my goodness, I hardly had to touch it!"

Well, he quickly became obsessed with pulling it out. When I changed clothes after church, I had hair ALL OVER my shirt. I was shedding like crazy. Hunter got the lint brush and cleaned all the hair off of my shirt!

At my aunt's after church, he had fun showing everyone just how easy it was to pull my hair out! Yeah - we are THAT family. No apologies!

I wanted to be sure to get a few pics of us together before the inevitable happens. We took a few pics out in the yard today. We were looking pretty sharp if I say so myself!

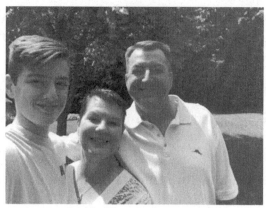

A pic of us before my hair is all gone!

So we have these great friends......and the husband is a barber. He's told me all along that whenever I was ready, he would be happy to shave my hair for me. I told him today at church that "it's about time!" His response was "just let me know." If he is anything - he is accommodating......and caring......and truly the FUNNIEST person I know. There's no way that shaving my head would NOT be an epic event if he was involved! And if you're gonna do it - it may as well be EPIC, right?!!!

As it turns out, he was going to the shop tonight to cut his kids hair.....and was kind enough to pencil me in as well. Lord, please don't let me have an ugly noggin', cause George will NEVER let me live it down! :-) George, Lisa and their sons Jake and Jackson were there with me, CC and Hunter. Just for the record - everybody needs friends like these guys.....I'm so very thankful to have them in my life and I feel blessed to have them supporting me through his adventure!

George got me all ready and gave Hunter some instructions on how to make the first swipe! Hunter buzzed off the first strips of hair! That was pretty cool!

George took over and went to work. My sweet friend Allie insisted that she thought I could rock a mohawk.......so just for you Allie B, George hooked me up with a temporary mohawk

We took lots of photos, videos with lively commentary - and as I imagined, it was ANYTHING but a sad time. We laughed and joked and poked fun. Jackson even said "that looks slick Mrs. Sonja" - and I just laughed out loud and said "pun intended, huh?"

So......late on a Sunday night.....18 days after my first chemo treatment I shaved my head. It just seemed like the wise thing to do. I came home tonight and took a shower to get cleaned up. Well - that was interesting! I realized that I have officially cut my shower time in half! No hair to wash and condition..........and no need to shave my underarms and legs anymore......so there is an unexpected joy bomb for ya!

And here we have it.......my hot-off-the-press new hair do.......or "no hair" do! A big shout out to the Evans family for making this a fun night for us! You guys are the best! We love ya'll to pieces! Bad jokes and all! :-)

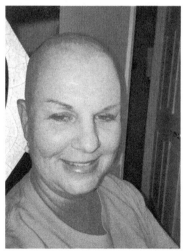

Rocking that fresh shaved look

So most days, I struggle finding just the right verse to share with my blog. I always want it to be relatable to the topic of the day. Well, today the verse came first - it seemed like a no-brainer to me! It seemed fitting that Luke 12:7 be the verse to accompany this post!

Praying for a great week. Chemo #2 coming up on Wednesday.

Blessings,

Sonja

Luke 12:7 The Message (MSG)
⁶⁻⁷ *What's the price of two or three pet canaries? Some loose change, right? But God never overlooks a single one. And he pays even greater attention to you, down to the last detail—even numbering the hairs on your head! So don't be intimidated by all this bully talk. You're worth more than a million canaries.*

SECOND TIME AROUND
July 19, 2017

Monday and Tuesday of this week were nothing short of WONDERFUL days.......I felt great, had lots of energy and was able to get some things done. It felt great to be able to run errands by myself if I chose. And as much as I was thankful for the two really great days this week, it was also a reminder to me that today, we started all over again. Today was chemo treatment day #2. But they say that's intentional spacing the infusion dates 3 weeks apart - you feel good for a few days after, then the next week is not so great, then the second week things start picking up......little more energy, feeling more like my old self........they don't want you coming in for your infusion when you are not feeling well. I know there is always a method to this madness.

I had lab work done at 9, dr appt at 9:30. The doctor's appt was running a little late, but we had a nice cushion of time between the dr appt and my chemo appointment. When the doctor was finally able to see me - we had a great visit - and I was all set to do chemo today. That's the reason for the blood work, so they can tell if your counts are where they need to be.

I told the medical oncologist today she was right on target with her estimate of when I'd lose my hair. She had said 10-12 days.......mine lasted a few days longer.

My exam with the medical oncologist was good. Nothing to worry about. Praise God!

After my doctor's appointment, we grabbed some lunch at Chick-Fil-A and then met my cousin at Duke North waiting area. She is a Life Flight nurse. She was all dressed like an astronaut!! We went upstairs to check out her work area, meeting coworkers and exploring the helipad.

My cousin gave us a tour of the Life Flight area and introduced us to some of the members of her team. This was her lifelong dream and she worked hard and it's paid off! So happy for her to truly be living her dream!

I had some time to kill after my doctor's appointment, so I went to the Belk Boutique and purchased a few more hats. I tried to get some "neutral" colors this time! The folks in the Belk Boutique are so kind and helpful. I always enjoy going in there.

Next up - Infusion Room. I was late getting started with chemo today b/c they were running 45 mins to 1 hr behind. My treatment takes 3 hours - so we were there a while. Everything went well with the chemo today (Praise the Lord)! No complications or anything. They also put on the Neulasta OnPro on my arm before I left. It will self-administer the meds around 9:00 pm tomorrow night.

Praying for no difficulties, fevers, chills, etc.

So last week, a friend was texting me saying we needed to get together to chat. She said she had some things going on in her life that she'd like to bounce off of me to get a fresh perspective. Well, almost immediately she text back and said - I can't do that to you. Why would you want to be bothered with my trivial mess with all you have going on?

I replied to her that I would WELCOME to chat with her about her concerns. I told her that just because I had cancer didn't mean that had to be the subject of every conversation. I reminded her that I LOVE to talk about things OTHER than this cancer. So she would be doing me a favor by sharing her concerns with me! You can vent to me anytime!!! Folks, I enjoy talking about my cancer experience.......but not EVERY DAY! If any of you have problems you may be facing, I'm here to listen!

So here's to being 2 treatments down.....and 10 more to go. Please pray they continue to be as uneventful as the first two!

It's been a long day.......and I keep dozing off trying to finish this......so I'm going to call it a night.

Have a great week!

Blessings,

Sonja

Psalm 118:24 New Living Translation (NLT)
[24] *This is the day the Lord has made. We will rejoice and be glad in it.*

JUST AN UPDATE
July 21, 2017

Well, Round #2 of chemo was pretty uneventful. I felt fine that evening and even the next morning. We had several things we needed to get done out of town and I even felt like taking care of business on Thursday. I lasted awhile - then I got really tired.....but thankfully we got all of our business taken care of without any complications.

I take a lot of flack because I'm a "mini-van mom." Apparently it isn't "cool" to drive a mini-van. I'll be honest, when I was in my early 20's, driving into the church parking lot one Sunday and seeing all the mini-vans there.........I remember saying, "Lord, please don't ever let me drive a mini-van!"

Fast forward many years after the birth of my son - all it took was one trip to the beach in a cramped Volvo S80 to change my opinion. I've driven a mini-van since 2004 and my son is now 14 and honestly......I can't imagine driving anything else. I'm 5'9" and officially the shortest person in the family. It takes a lottttt of leg room for this family. And talk about storage! It's enough room in there for us and all of our STUFF!

Yesterday on the way home, I was so very thankful for my mini-van. I sat in the 2nd row of seats and reclined them and I was able to stretch out and relax and get some sleep on the way home. No shame here!

After we got home, I laid down awhile just to rest.

Thankfully, we had some great friends bring us dinner last night. It was such a blessing not to have to worry about dinner for my family. I had a great appetite and was able to enjoy the meal. That is always a plus!

Today, I woke up feeling fine. I have to eat as soon as I get up so I can start taking my meds. That is still one of the worst things for me - I am NOT a fan of eating as soon as I get up and I'm definitely not one to wake up early just so I can wait awhile to eat and take my medicine! :-) Afterwards, I was able to write some checks, get them mailed and run by the bank and that little run of energy slap wore me out. I came home and took a 2 hour nap after only being up 3 hours. That's crazy how it can just jump on you like that. I honestly think I could nap right now but I surely don't want to be up all night!

Nothing really tastes good today.....soups and fruits tend to be my "go-to" foods but even some days they don't taste good. So if you ask me at lunch what sounds good for dinner - well, chances are whatever sounds good at lunch will taste like crap by the time dinner rolls around. But....I keep trying to eat SOMETHING just because I know I need to.

Praying this will pass quickly - but all in all - I am doing well. These hiccups are to be expected, and I think the best thing I can do is listen to my body and praise God for the strength to get through each day with whatever challenges the day brings. So far, He has not let me down - and I don't anticipate that He will.

This morning - within about 30 mins of each other - I had two friends send me this song. That's not coincidence, my friends. Find and listen to *I'm Gonna Love You Through It* when you get a moment - it's an awesome song and a great inspiration to me and many others fighting this nasty disease. I've been blessed with having "my tribe" of friends and family near and far loving me through this mess.....and I will never, ever be able to adequately express how much I appreciate all of you who have shown up in so many different ways. Bringing food, sending cards, texts, meals, transportation, prayers.......Saying "thank you" just doesn't seem to be enough.

God sends us just what we need......in just the right time. I needed to hear *I'm Gonna Love You Through It* today and I'm thankful for you two ladies who shared this with me! Thanks Diane and Ginny!

Wishing each of you a safe, happy and blessed week end.

Blessings,

Sonja

Job 2:11 New Life Version (NLV)
[11] *Now when Job's three friends heard of all this trouble that had come upon him, they came each from his own place. They were Eliphaz the Temanite, Bildad the Shuhite, and Zophar the Naamathite. They agreed to meet together to come to share Job's sorrow and comfort him.*

COMMUNITY
July 7, 2017

Our message at church this morning was on "Created for Community." Pastor Karl reminded us that Jesus created us for community and that God has said for us to be alone is NOT a good thing. He wants us to be one with Him and one with each other.

This message was especially meaningful for me today. Since my cancer diagnosis, I've experienced the love and blessings of "community" from my church, my family, my friends, even from random strangers. I've "heard" about community and thought I understood the impact of community - but honestly, I don't think I ever truly "got" it until now.

I understood it from the "giving" end, but being on the receiving end of so many acts of love, kindness and compassion has been overwhelming, but very humbling. It has shown me a real glimpse of what being the hands and feet of Jesus truly is about. One of the biggest lessons I've learned is how important it is to be honest when folks ask you "what do you need" or "what can I do for you?" They are being sincere in asking - and it's important that I be honest in my response. So often we just brush things off and say, "oh, I'm fine, I don't need anything" when in fact there very well may be something we do need, and when we don't express that need to others, we are robbing them of THEIR blessing.

Think about that for a minute. They are asking because they truly want to give and truly want to show us love in ways big and small. It would be such a shame for us to rob them of their ability to BLESS us when we are in need.

So this week, when I had friends ask what they could do for me or bring me - I simply said "soup." Soup has consistently been the one thing that seems to always taste good.

So this week I was blessed immensely by my "community" with chicken 'n dumplings, vegetable soup, wonton soup, chicken and rice soup and good ole' potato soup. They asked - I gave them an honest answer - and we ALL were blessed. That wasn't so difficult, was it?

Well, sometimes it can seem difficult to "ask" for help - but it gets easier - I promise. When you realize it is a win-win for you and the person offering the help - it makes it so much easier to put yourself out there. Go on, give it a try! I know you will be blessed! :-)

Pastor Karl also reminded us to share with those in need and to practice hospitality. I can honestly say that my "community" sharing with me and showing me so much hospitality has blessed me immensely. It's been nothing short of amazing.

Last night I got a text from a college roommate asking me what would be a good day for her to come and visit and bring me her famous sesame chicken potato salad. I quickly responded what days were available. While I'm sure her dish will be delicious - I'm even more excited that she's willing to drive 3 hours to see me and just come and lift my spirits. What a "joy bomb."

Today, riding home from church, I got a message from a friend just saying she was praying for me and that God would get me through this and offered support whether I needed to laugh, cry or just vent! Another "joy bomb!" God keeps continuing to bless me and my family in ways I could never have imagined.

My son asked me a few minutes ago if we had any plans for next week because he had a sweet friend who had texted to say she wanted to take him out to lunch one day just to get him out of the house. I CANNOT tell you how much that meant to me.

God uses the young and old alike.

How awesome that this young girl felt compelled to reach out to my kid! My heart was about to explode. Trying to give him as much normalcy as possible during all of this has been my biggest concern.

I can't take this cancer away, but he sure deserves to "get away" from this cancer from time to time! What may have seemed like just a small gesture to this young friend, was a HUGE blessing to this mama bear.

And I've gotta say - I'm embracing this whole "bald" thing. Lawd - it is so "freeing." No hair to wash, dry, style......no hair products to purchase. I never imagined I'd embrace it this much. So much so that I entertained visitors yesterday in my baldness.

It is what it is.

Be prepared - if you stop by, you are likely to catch me without a cap or scarf on. The only thing that would make it better is if I had a bit of "color" on my noggin. It's pretty dang pasty white!

I purchased a wig a few weeks ago. I decided I needed to "name" it. I opted for "Stella" (from the movie Stella Got Her Groove Back).

Yeah - this cancer may have got me sidetracked for a bit - but just you wait - I'm gonna get my groove back too!

Each day that passes is one day closer to me being done with this treatment and crossing the finish line with a happy, healthy future. Just you wait!

Hugs,

Sonja

(I admit I'm stealing my "verse of the day" today from Pastor Karl's sermon. But it truly says it all.)

Romans 12:9-15 New International Version (NIV)
⁹ Love must be sincere. Hate what is evil; cling to what is good. ¹⁰ Be devoted to one another in love. Honor one another above yourselves. ¹¹ Never be lacking in zeal, but keep your spiritual fervor, serving the Lord. ¹² Be joyful in hope, patient in affliction, faithful in prayer. ¹³ Share with the Lord's people who are in need. Practice hospitality. ¹⁴ Bless those who persecute you; bless and do not curse. ¹⁵ Rejoice with those who rejoice; mourn with those who mourn.

FINDING A PATTERN
July 26, 2017

The weird thing about chemo (at least for me) has been that the "after effects" don't show up right away. My chemo treatments have been given on Wednesdays - and typically, Thurs/Fri/Sat/Sun are pretty "normal" - maybe a little more tired than usual.....but still pretty normal as far as feeling good. I've tried to be diligent about keeping up with good days and bad days on the calendar - trying to see if there is any method to the madness or any distinct patterns.

I think I can confidently say that I have noticed a pattern to the Mondays after chemo.........those days are certifiably CRAPPY (pun intended - queue the CRAP emoji)!

I've had two treatments and both Mondays after chemo were NO FUN. Both times I was plagued with diarrhea......Imodium is my new best friend on Mondays after chemo! I was so weak - all I had the energy to do was lay around and nap off and on all day.

I thought I'd feel like I would have energy enough to do a simple task around the house......BUT NO!!! You feel like you "need" to do something or want to push yourself just a bit thinking if you just get up and get going, it'll get better - but it JUST.......DOESN'T..... HAPPEN!

Sunday I felt great......went to church, out for lunch, came home and napped, took Hunter to the lake for a youth outing......and felt WONDERFUL the entire time! How can so much change overnight? I don't know but it sure does! I think I slept most of the day on Monday and finally at 9ish - I said the heck with this, I'm going to bed. My body just ached. Ugh - enough of this all ready!

What a difference a day makes! Thankfully - Tuesday was sooooo much better! Now I didn't wake up feeling like I could run a marathon - but I did wake up without a queasy stomach - and that's always a plus. Those mornings when you literally put your feet on the floor and the nausea hits - they are awful! I'm learning that I need to "ease" myself into things! Like having a cup of coffee.....letting my stomach settle and trying to eat some breakfast maybe an hour later. Showers don't typically happen first thing in the mornings any more.........it may be mid-late afternoon or even after dinner.

Whatever works, right? It just all depends on the day.

Sometimes you just need to get up and get out and get some fresh air - but honestly, the "getting there" can seem so difficult sometimes, you just say the heck with it. And it's been so incredibly hot here - this heat sucks the life out of you when you feel good - much less when you're tackling chemo!

But I celebrate that Tuesday was a better day and today is even better than yesterday! Small steps.......and yes it is important to celebrate the small things! And honestly - if Mondays after chemo are the worst days I have to endure - then I have very little to complain about! In the grand scheme of things - I've been very blessed to not be sick, throwing up, dehydrated, running fevers, etc. I count it a blessing that my side effects have been minimal and truly feel a bit guilty for complaining.

And in other good news - CC was released from the doctor to return to work this week. Praise God he is doing better - he had quite a tough go of it for a while. While we are both thankful that he is doing well enough to return to work - it was bittersweet for me. We had been home together for over a month.......and I admit, it was nice having him here "just in case." It will be an adjustment having him gone - but I still have my sidekick here for a few more weeks to keep me company and take care of me!

It's amazing how God works in the background - while it was unfortunate CC was home with a herniated disc and in immense pain, it was a blessing to have him here with me during this time. God knows our needs.......and gives us just what we need in just the right time.

So I've had lots of information shared with me since my diagnosis about so many cancer support groups, networks, organizations, etc. I thought it would make sense to share some of these sites here in case others may be able to benefit from them as well.

Hope Abounds provides supportive services, financial assistance, educational opportunities and advocacy for women, children, teens and their families, who are going through any type of cancer from diagnosis to survivorship.

www.hopeabounds.org

Cleaning for a Reason is an awesome organization. Unfortunately, it isn't currently available in my rural area - but it may be available near you. Please share with anyone you may know who may be able to benefit from this wonderful service!

http://cleaningforareason.org

https://breastcancerfreebies.com

A friend shared these two links with me for great options for eyebrows and eyelashes (since they disappear also with chemo). I'll definitely be ordering these eyebrow kits!

And wouldn't you know - I had just finished a round of Rodan + Fields Lash Boost just before my diagnosis and my eyelashes were

AHHMAZING if I say so myself.......and now I'm just waiting to see how long they stay around. Oh well - it's just eye lashes. If they don't grow back - lillylashes.com has some rocking ones!

http://www.anastasiabeverlyhills.com/beauty-express/abh-beauty-express.html?cgid=fillers#sz=12&start=14&cgid=fillers

https://lillylashes.com/?gclid=CI7z0KvT0tQCFYc2gQodkDgEhA

So I initially wrote the bulk of this blog last night and hoped to publish it then - but I was really tired, and I just didn't feel good about it and I finally decided I would just save it and finish it today. I didn't want to make a hasty decision on a quote, content or Bible verse......so I closed my laptop and said I'll tackle that tomorrow.

Well....just so you know - that was God prompting me.

This morning, I got an email from a friend from church - her emails are ALWAYS so encouraging and bring a smile to my face. You'd never know that her own family is going through their own personal health storms.......she's quite amazing. But her email this morning indicated she wanted to share some scripture with me.

No doubt this was God's handiwork. This was one of the verses that she shared and it is just PERFECT to accompany this post.
God never......ever.....disappoints! He's there on the good days and the crappy days!

Blessings,

Sonja

James 1:2 New International Version (NIV)
[2] *Consider it pure joy, my brothers and sisters, whenever you face trials of many kinds.*

NO MORE 3 X 5'S
July 27, 2017

We live in a world of instant everything. I got my first digital camera before my son was born 14 years ago; I have no idea just how many pictures I have taken of him over the years. Now, we hardly ever use a real "camera" because the camera quality on our phones is amazing. We take pictures to "document" everything. First day of school, birthdays, dinner out with friends, food.....you get the picture (pun intended). We are all so busy trying to "capture" the perfect moments in a picture that.......well......we are not truly living in the moment and enjoying the moment for all it's worth........and I believe we are doing ourselves a huge injustice.

Yesterday I was emailing back and forth with a friend whose husband has been going through his own health crisis for the last several years. With everything she has going on in her own corner of the world......she has consistently checked in on me via email, Facebook, cards or gifts sent in the mail. She is an encourager......and she truly uses her "gift" of encouraging others. I'm so blessed to have her as a friend and so very thankful to have her in my life.

Anyway - in our email conversations, I mentioned how having a "diagnosis" changes you. Instantly. Here's an excerpt from the email I sent her......

> As you guys know - a cancer diagnosis changes you instantly. It changes your outlook, perspective, how you view simple things in every day life. It makes you appreciate more, and let things that used to upset you roll off your back. A night at home with your family on the couch watching mindless TV is a beautiful thing. You just enjoy being in the moment.
>
> I often think of a song by John Mayer called 3x5. We're such a generation of capturing everything on camera - but I'm finding myself enjoying the "moment" now - just capturing it on my brain and in my heart - and not capturing it in print on a photograph.

and here's how she responded......

> These days I find myself capturing special moments and will remember them forever. Funny you mention sitting on the couch at night watching TV; that is exactly what we do. So many tasks have been neglected, but I would not take anything for spending time with him each evening doing nothing, but enjoying being together.

For those of you who may not be familiar with the John Mayer song, 3x5, here's a link to a YouTube video with the lyrics.

https://www.youtube.com/watch?v=GP5gWbyuXrs

I encourage you to take a few minutes and listen to the song and truly think about the words. This song has been placed on my heart for awhile now - and some of the lyrics that speak to me the most are these:

Didn't have a camera by my side this time. Hoping I would see the world with both my eyes/ You should have seen that sunrise with your own eyes. It brought me back to /Today I finally overcame/ Trying to fit the world inside a picture frame

Most of us are all guilty of rushing through life - and maybe trying to capture our moments and experiences in a photo or video - but how often do we really stop and just try to soak up the moment.......to live IN that moment and just totally take it all in.....the sights, the sounds, the smells, the emotions. I can tell you this - hearing the word "cancer" has made me much more aware of these things. And yes - I still take pictures from time to time - but I'm much more inclined to stop and soak up the sights and sounds from my back porch on a summer night..........or sit in the swing on a stormy day and enjoy the feel of the wind on my bald head.......or watch the expression in my son's eyes when he figures out a difficult task......or feel thankful for the "crowded" bed when all 3 of us pile in to watch NCIS reruns.......or enjoy the sound of laughter from two teenage boys in the backseat of the car.

When we try to "fit the world inside a picture frame" - we truly lose out on so much.

Am I a little sad that my college roommate drove 3 hours to see me yesterday and we got so carried away catching up that I forgot to take a picture of us? Well......yeah. But.....for the time that she was here - we were able to immerse ourselves in each other.......yakking it up on the couch.......just like when were 18 back at UNCG. It was as if we picked up right where we left off. I have the memory of yesterday tucked away in a very special place in my heart and imprinted on my brain! No 3x5 needed.

Today was an awesome day - Hunter and I were able to go out and do something "fun" for a change. We went to Raleigh to an "Escape Room." If you have never tried them, they are really cool and a lot of fun (and super frustrating all at the same time). Hunter's friend and his mom went with us and the four us had a lot of laughs trying to figure out the clues to solve the mystery and "Escape" the room before the one hour time limit. The Escape Room did not allow cell phones - so there were no pictures taken. But I spent an hour just enjoying the experience. We struggled......we got frustrated......we kept at it.....and we made some great memories......and YES - we did escape with literally seconds left! We were all intrigued and anxious to try another one soon!

So my advice to you is this: stop trying to fit the world inside a picture frame......and take time to see the world with your OWN eyes. Live "in" the moment! I'm pretty sure you will be pleasantly surprised. Sometimes you just need to relax, breathe and just live in the moment!

I challenge each of you to make an effort to truly "live" in the moment over the next few days. When you feel compelled to reach for your phone to take a picture........stop and rethink it........and just enjoy the moment in real time.

Be blessed!

Sonja

Ephesians 5:15-16 New International Version (NIV)
[15] *Be very careful, then, how you live—not as unwise but as wise,* [16] *making the most of every opportunity, because the days are evil.*

IT HAPPENS FOR A REASON
July 30, 2017

Well I've had several great days in a row - and I praise God for them! You quickly learn to celebrate each and every victory - whether big or small.

Friday I was able to go with my mom to Danville for a bit. While we were out and about, we stopped by Subway to grab a bite to eat. Since it was so hot, I opted to leave "Stella" at home and just wore a red bandana on my head. As we were in line at Subway placing our order, the young manager looked at me and asked if I was going through chemo. I smiled and said yes, then asked him if my hairdo gave it away. He just smiled and said yes and told me that he had a cousin who went through chemo and then he said "your sandwich is on me today."

Can I tell you that I have shed a handful of tears since I was diagnosed with cancer - which is nothing short of a miracle for those of you who know me well. I can ONLY attribute it to the good Lord sustaining me (my buddy Zeke will confirm I can cry "on demand" if you have any doubts)......but let me tell you that in that moment as the manager said those words, I became a blubbering mess. The tears just WOULD. NOT. STOP.

I tried to say "thank you" - but it took me a good while to recover myself to even get the words out. I was so taken by surprise and just so amazed at a complete stranger's random act of kindness. It's crazy what can tug right at your heart strings. And the amazing thing is - we were torn between going to Subway and Sonic. I wanted a Cherry Limeade from Sonic, but I knew mom liked Subway - and there was an ETERNAL line at Sonic and last time we were there, it was a short line and it still took FOREVER - so last minute I opted for us to just go to Subway. God was steering us there the entire time. He was steering me in the direction of an unexpected blessing (or "joy bomb"). He is always right on time. I doubt that manager has any idea just how much he blessed me that day.

Sundays are always good days. We attended church today and that's always a blessing. Awesome people, wonderful message, and great fellowship.

As I stated above, I am......by nature......an extremely tender-hearted person and can cry on demand.....always have been. I've been completely amazed at myself and how well I have handled and accepted this cancer diagnosis. Me handling this "so well" as many have said has been totally out of character for me.

Two years ago, I began training at church for Stephen Ministry. It's a one-on-one distinctively Christian care ministry. Stephen Ministers provide confidential, Christ-centered care to people who are hurting (illness, grief, divorce, job loss, etc). There's a link below for more information. If you don't have this ministry in your church, I would urge you to look into it. It has been a blessing for our church and the Stephen Ministers and the Care Receivers all!

http://www.stephenministries.org

Certification for Stephen Ministry requires 50 hours of training. It's long and intensive - but I can tell you that the training I received as a Stephen Minister has benefited me in my own life. Literally the day after I became commissioned as a Stephen Minister, my husband's brother passed away very unexpectedly. My husband lost his brother and his very best friend all at once. While I wasn't prepared to put my training into practice so quickly, the Stephen Ministry training regarding caring for those who are grieving was an INVALUABLE tool for me during that time. It helped me better understand what my husband was going through, that he was allowed to "feel" however he felt - and to know that the grieving process is different for every person. Again - God's timing was perfect.

Fast forward a few years to my cancer diagnosis……again, the training I received helped me to understand not just my own feelings regarding the diagnosis, but to understand that processing this diagnosis would be different for me and my husband, my child and my parents and family. While I thought my training was simply going to be for me to help others in their times of need - it turned I needed that training every bit as much for myself for the events that would unfold in our lives over the next few years. **Everything happens for a reason.**

Last year I also attended The Walk to Emmaus. Our church is a strong supporter of The Walk to Emmaus and we have quite a number of folks who have attended this life-transforming weekend. It's a wonderful spiritual retreat……72 hours spent worshipping, learning, reflecting, singing, and participating in small groups. It's a weekend filled with Christian love in action. You simply CANNOT leave The Walk unchanged. My friend Zeke had told me "just like the 2 men in the Bible, YOU WILL encounter Jesus on your walk."…..and he was right.

While they were talking and discussing, Jesus himself came near and walked with them." - Luke 24:15

It was truly one of those "mountain top" experiences for me. The Walk to Emmaus is sponsored by The Upper Room and is open to any Christian denomination. If your church is not participating in The Walk to Emmaus, I strongly urge you to consider learning more about this wonderful weekend! You won't regret it!

http://emmaus.upperroom.org/about

So to answer the question "how am I doing so well" handling this diagnosis. I am quite certain that the Stephen Ministry training and my Walk To Emmaus weekend were two things that DEFINITELY happened for a reason.

Each of these experiences helped deepen my walk with Christ, introduced me to some wonderful Christian friends and mentors........and I am confident these experiences left me better prepared to handle the curve ball I was thrown on May 1, 2017. God was working in the background to prepare me mentally, emotionally and spiritually. Now that doesn't mean that I am implying this has all been easy. It surely hasn't.

I've had my ups and downs - but the downs have definitely been few. I have also had an enormous amount of folks near and far lifting me in prayer on a daily basis. I have felt those prayers and I am so thankful for each and every prayer warrior who has interceded on my behalf.

God has definitely blessed this mess......time and time again. While I know I'm on the front end of this adventure.......there may be some long, difficult days ahead. But I am confident that the same God who has worked to prepare me for this season in my life will continue to walk beside me......step by step......day by day.......minute by minute and help me cross the finish line. Of that......I am certain.

Lastly - I feel I must take a moment to say "thank you" to so many of you who have reached out to me regarding my blog. I admit - this is a first for me. I've never "blogged" before.....and while I felt like I was "doing this for me" - I'm learning that many others are benefitting from my blog as well. How can that be?

I am completely in awe that so many have even read my blog and honestly had no idea that my words would ever have the "reach" that it has. That can only be attributed to the good Lord. I just felt compelled to share my story......He gets credit for the rest. And I must say when I've received texts saying "I had my mammogram this week" or "I've scheduled my FIRST EVER mammogram."......well, that is exactly why I'm doing this! Prevention is key my friends!

Be blessed! Have a great week!

Hugs!

Sonja

Ecclesiastes 3:11 New International Version (NIV)
[11] *He has made everything beautiful in its time. He has also set eternity in the human heart; yet no one can fathom what God has done from beginning to end.*

PUSHING THROUGH
August 1, 2017

Monday was one of those "I feel so normal, how can I possibly have cancer" days. I felt great, had TONS of energy......ran a few errands in town and even cooked dinner. The weather last night was PERFECT back porch weather. I had to MAKE myself go in at bedtime.....I was truly enjoying sitting outside, listening to the sounds of nature......and enjoying the nice breeze. It doesn't get much better than that! :-)

Once I could no longer hold my eyes open.......I reluctantly went inside and went to bed. CC was not feeling well yesterday and appeared to be coming down with a cold (or better known around here as "the MAN flu."...Google it - it's a thing). Because I am so FEARFUL of catching ANYTHING due to my compromised immune system......I slept in the spare bedroom last night. One can't be too cautious! I love him, but I don't want whatever he's got!

I woke up around 6 am this morning and used the potty and went right back to bed. The next thing I know - I woke up and looked at the clock.......it was 10:15am. Holy smokes Batman! What in the world?? I struggled even then to focus on the clock - my eyes were stuck together I had slept so hard. You would think I would have felt like I could conquer the world after a night of sleep like that.....but I. JUST. COULDN'T. wake up. A shower ALWAYS works. NOT TODAY! I literally felt like I could fall asleep at a moments notice all day long. I didn't feel AWFUL, but I didn't feel great at all. Total 180 degrees from the day I had yesterday. That HAS to be the most difficult thing for me to wrap my brain around about all this. How you can go from 0-60 mph in no time flat? I don't know......but you can.

Today was the first day I really felt like I had to PUSH THROUGH and just not give in. I just felt "different" today. And....1) I don't **like** not feeling good and...2) I don't like **admitting** that I don't feel good. I really do try to be a glass half full kinda person.

I was afraid if I slept all day (which I'm confident I could have) that I would have been up all night - and then that just creates a vicious cycle. I busied myself with anything just to keep from going to bed and sleeping the day away. We even gave Bella a MUCH needed bath (she probably wished I had chosen to take a nap).....but we can't have a stinking dog around here!

So now that we've made it past dinner (thanks BJ for the peas and corn and the peach preserves were awesome Janis!)......I'm back out on the porch....to enjoy this wonderful weather again for a little bit before calling it night.

I guess our bodies know what we need - and apparently I had run a little low on sleep. I wonder if the cooler temperatures helped me sleep more soundly? I dunno. I hope and pray I sleep as good tonight......but I do hope I wake up more "alert" tomorrow than I was today!

But either way......I'm thankful......thankful for God's blessings on me on days when I feel like crap. Thankful that I didn't have to worry about dinner for my crew - BJ took care of that for me......thankful that my guys are understanding that somedays mom just is not at her best. There's still SOOOOO much to be thankful for.

I'm sure this won't be the only day that pushing through will be a challenge.....I feel sure there will be many more "not-so-great days" along this ride.......but having days like today make days like YESTERDAY all the more precious......and I look forward to more good days than bad.

Man....I really hate to leave this back porch again.....thank you Lord for this perfect weather!

Nite!

Sonja

Psalm 18:32 New International Version (NIV)
[32] *It is God who arms me with strength and keeps my way secure.*

YOU'VE GOT MAIL!
August 5, 2017

My Grandma Blanks had many great qualities - but one of the things she was "best" known for was sending get well cards. If you were sick (or even had a cold) - you could COUNT ON receiving a card from my grandma. It's been a running joke in our family that if the preacher announced on Sunday that you were having surgery on Wednesday.......well, chances were good that the get well card would arrive at the hospital before you did. Grandma didn't drive......so she couldn't hop in the car and come visit you.......but she could write.....and sending a card was her way of witnessing to folks. Sending cards was truly her gift. Lordy, I just wonder how many cards she sent over the years. It was thousands I'm sure! And those card boxes were recycled too.....we'd receive our Christmas gifts in them each year! Grandma didn't waste much!

There was a time.......before I became a mom......that I was good about sending cards (NEVER great about it like my grandma, just GOOD). I joke that all my organizational skills came out with the placenta as soon as I gave birth. I often have the best of intentions......but I just never have gotten back on track sending cards like I once did. I guess life just happens.

Thankfully - it is not a lost art for MANY! I have been completely overwhelmed at the number of cards I have received since my diagnosis. The cards come in spurts. There may be a day when there are 5+ in the mailbox......and then none for a few days.....and then they will trickle in again. But what I can tell you is THIS......those cards arrive JUST. AT. THE. PERFECT. TIME. It's not random!

Some days, it's a verse or quote on a card that really speaks to me......and other times, it's simply the person that sent it to me. I've received cards from folks I didn't even know that really knew me (and maybe they don't) - but they sent me a card anyway!

And I've also received cards from folks who have their own share of struggles.....but they find time to send me a card to wish me well. Then there's the cards from cancer survivors who give me encouragement to keep my head up and keep fighting. Sometimes it's a card from someone I haven't seen or talked to in FOREVER.

Shortly after I found out I had cancer - two childhood friends (also breast cancer survivors) came over one night and brought this tub filled with food. The food went away quickly - but the tub quickly became my "collection spot" for my cards. This tub stays in the window seat in my kitchen. I'm able to keep them all in one place - but I love having them sitting out as a visual reminder of how many folks have encouraged me and are praying for me! I can sit down and re-read them whenever I want.

Then there's some that get to adorn the refrigerator......because that's what you do when a sweet young fella makes you a work of art!

And let's NOT discount social media.......texting........or visiting. Not everyone has a gift of sending cards - but MANY have kept in touch with me and wished me well through Facebook, or texting, calling or visiting. Many mornings I wake up and have an unread text waiting for me from someone that simply says they're thinking of me and wanted to share certain scripture with me.

Those texts always arrive at just the right time - maybe it was a difficult morning or I wasn't feeling my best. And I'll never forget the morning of June 28th, when I was standing in line to check in at the lab at the cancer center on my first day of chemo. As I stood there, I got a message on my phone from a breast cancer survivor saying they were thinking of me as I started my treatments and that I would be just fine......it was like God was winking at me saying, "I've got this."

So many have come by to sit and chat and catch up.......and I so enjoy your visits! Some just pop in for a quick minute or two and some stay for hours and I'm thankful for each and every visitor. Laughter is always good for the soul - and your visits almost always are sure to promise lots of laughter. In our family - we're not real formal. No need to call before you come - just come on over any time! Just don't be shocked when you catch me with nothing on my head and make-up free!

Then there are those that have faithfully called me each week to check in to see how I've been doing. They may not always get me on the phone - and if they don't, they just leave a quick message to say they were calling to see how my week was going.

So - not everyone can be like Grandma Blanks. Sending cards is NOT everyone's gift. And that's just fine! My point is this - WHATEVER your gift is - **DO NOT DISCOUNT IT.**

You may think that sending a card or texting or calling or visiting or bringing food is "not such a big thing."…..but trust me - the recipient truly knows that "it is a big deal!"

I am happy to report that I have had 3 awesome days…..Wed/Thur/Fri could not have been better. I'm learning to make the most of the good days…..whenever they come around…….and take those ugly days like Tuesday to just be still and know that it's okay to do nothing.

So far - today seems to be a good one as well. Praise God! I'll take it!

I have been a little snotty the past few days - I hope I'm not coming down with anything. I feel okay - just my nose is a bit stuffy......that makes it a little difficult to sleep with my CPAP!

Lastly - I decided yesterday that I was tired of my head feeling like a big piece of Velcro.

Even though I had my head shaved with the clippers - and much of my hair had come out on its own - there was still this crazy stubble that was honestly, quite painful. They say the chemo causes your hair follicles to become inflamed - and when I would touch my head - it felt like pin pricks.

So yesterday, I marched into Community Barber Shop and told my friend George I needed him to shave my head. Yeah - I did that! I WILLINGLY gave George permission to take a straight razor to my head! What was I thinking?! Oh my - it was wonderful! That hot shaving cream on my bald head felt soooooo good!

I was turned away from the mirror, so I couldn't see what George was doing (probably a good thing)! But I survived okay!

Let me just tell you that my noggin is as smooth as a baby's bottom! No more pin pricks! I'm telling ya'll - this bald thing ain't so bad!

Wonder if George needs a new spokesmodel for Community Barber Shop? Wonder how much it pays?

Have a great weekend!

Be blessed!

Sonja

(So I loved both of these versions of 1 Peter 4:10 - so I had to share them both.)

1 Peter 4:10 New International Version (NIV)
[10] Each of you should use whatever gift you have received to serve others, as faithful stewards of God's grace in its various forms.

1 Peter 4:10-11 The Message (MSG)
[7-11] Everything in the world is about to be wrapped up, so take nothing for granted. Stay wide-awake in prayer. Most of all, love each other as if your life depended on it. Love makes up for practically anything. Be quick to give a meal to the hungry, a bed to the homeless—cheerfully. Be generous with the different things God gave you, passing them around so all get in on it: if words, let it be God's words; if help, let it be God's hearty help. That way, God's bright presence will be evident in everything through Jesus, and he'll get all the credit as the One mighty in everything—encores to the end of time. Oh, yes!

MY CURRENT SITUATION
August 7, 2017

Well......you knew it had to happen.....eventually. Saturday morning as I typed my last blog entry, I was feeling really good. I was a little snotty - but that was okay. Fast forward to around 3 pm on Saturday and I truly felt like I had been hit by a truck. I could hardly hold my eyes open. I took some Tylenol and went to bed around 3:30 and slept for a few hours. Woke up still feeling not so great - and Hunter and I laid in my bed watching a Hallmark movie (yeah - he hates 'em, and loves to go ahead and tell me after the first 5 minutes just how it's gonna end - MEN - they just don't get it!).

Being the great helper that he is......he volunteered to help me get supper ready. He truly is handy in the kitchen! I felt a little better after dinner and we started working on a puzzle. If you hafta feel like crap and be stuck at home - you may as well make the most of it, right?

I didn't sleep well Saturday night and was sniffling and sneezing most of the night. We talked the night before and everyone seemed to feel like it would be in my best interest if I DIDN'T go to church on Sunday if I was still feeling yucky. I surely didn't need to risk making things worse or picking up any germs. Well - given that I didn't wake up Sunday til around 9:30 - it's safe to say I didn't make it to church. I laid around the house all day Sunday trying to shake whatever was trying to jump on me.

My biggest fear is that I might catch ANYTHING that may prevent me from having my chemo on the assigned day. I'm a planner by nature - and if I put in my calendar - IT NEEDS TO HAPPEN ON THAT DAY!! Even though I have not been given an END DATE to my chemo treatments - I am MENTALLY checking them off my list. Right now we are at 2 down and 10 to go - with the next treatment being on Friday. It's written on the calendar - so it needs to happen! Right now - according to MY CALENDAR :-) I should finish up this first regimen on Wednesday, August 30th. I don't know how soon after that treatment that they will start me on the next regimen - which will be 8 treatments - once a week for 8 weeks. So it's difficult to know right now just when my last treatment will fall - it all depends on when they start me on the Taxol. I'd guess it's going to be mid to late November by the time I wrap this chemo up.....that is, if I don't have any delays.

That being said......this will surely put me in the middle of cold/flu season.......and let's not forget about the kids returning to school and sharing germs there......so when I start thinking of it in those terms - it makes me very concerned about staying healthy.

While it's probably NOT a great idea to go to Wal-Mart or places where there are A LOT of folks (translated TONS of germs).......it's difficult to think about staying at home ALL the time. While I've enjoyed being able to spend so much time this summer with Hunter while he's been out of school - at least I've been able to go grocery shopping or run to Wal-Mart when I needed to. After the past few days - I'm starting to wonder if I need to rethink that. Ugh - it's such a conundrum!!! And to top it off - my favorite sport season is upon us.......Volleyball.......I really don't want to miss those games! :-(

I plan to discuss this further with my doctor on Friday. There HAS to be a happy medium. I don't want to feel like I'm in solitary confinement! :-) But I don't want to delay my treatments either! This would probably be less of an issue if I were an introvert......however.....that's NOT the case!

I have to keep reminding myself that this is just TEMPORARY.....and that this, too, shall pass.

Enjoy this beautiful day! It's great for back porch sitting.....that's exactly where I am right now!

Blessings,

Sonja

Isaiah 41:10 The Message (MSG)
8-10 "But you, Israel, are my servant. You're Jacob, my first choice, descendants of my good friend Abraham. I pulled you in from all over the world, called you in from every dark corner of the earth, Telling you, 'You're my servant, serving on my side. I've picked you. I haven't dropped you.' Don't panic. I'm with you. There's no need to fear for I'm your God. I'll give you strength. I'll help you. I'll hold you steady, keep a firm grip on you."

GOOD DAYS AND BAD DAYS
August 10, 2017

Well......I'm happy to report that I have felt much better since Tuesday! Praise the Lord! Still snotty and sneezing like crazy and some body aches here and there (I'm assuming that's from the Lunesta injection I get each time after a chemo treatment).....but overall, much better than earlier this week.

And today has been a really good day (seems to be the case each time before the next treatment)! It's like it's timed just perfectly to psyche you out - to have you feeling pretty "normal" only to go in tomorrow for chemo round #3. But......I'm learning to make the most of the days I feel "normal."..... and just try to do very little and take care of myself on the not-so-good days. I always have a book (or three) handy - and there's always thank you cards to write.....so those are good options for the yucky days.....along with Hallmark movies (much to everyone else's dismay). And if laying around and sleeping is all I feel like doing - well, by golly, I've given myself permission to do just that!

My "normal" days this week allowed me to feel good enough to take Hunter to the orthodontist in Durham........two days in a row! This kid has held on to his baby teeth FOREVER and we couldn't get his braces til they were all gone. He had one tooth hanging on by a thread - so the orthodontist was able to pull it easily on Tuesday. After that - he said "we're ready for his braces now." Well, given the fact that he will start school next Thursday and my current health situation - I asked if there was any way we could get them put on before school started. Surprisingly, they said "sure, can you be here in the morning?" How could I refuse? I'm very thankful that I was able to accompany him to those appointments.

I'm glad I'm feeling good today......physically anyway......mentally, I'm having to wrap my brain around the fact that I will be attending HIGH SCHOOL Open House with my son tonight. HOW CAN THAT BE? It seems like only a few months ago that I walked him into school for kindergarten!! Time surely flies. He's grown into a wonderful young man right before my eyes. I have a feeling the next 4 years are going to go by even faster than the last 14.

We survived open house - I'm still in denial that my child is now a high schooler! But I learned tonight that I have lots of other folks in denial with me! Overall, I'm thankful for the great group of friends Hunter has......and one in particular......crazy Gavin. These two hit it off in 1st grade and have been thick as thieves since then. I love it also because it's not just a friendship between these two boys - but between both of our families. There is NEVER a dull moment with these two and you NEVER know what you will learn when you spend an hour or so with these cuties!

And can I just say a big "thank you" to all of you who have provided food for our family over the last several months. We have been so blessed to have so many delicious meals brought to us. Whether you cooked or brought take out or treated us out to dinner.....or secretly left tomatoes on the porch for us to make tomato sandwiches - we are eternally grateful. It's been great to be able to pull things out of the freezer on nights I didn't feel like cooking! Someone gave us a gift certificate to the new Rising Son Bakery here in town. We were able to use the gift certificate to purchase anything from either Rising Son or the Farm to Home Market......they had some frozen chicken pot pies and I got one of those to have on hand for a quick meal sometimes. I was happy to know that they offer gift certificates. I'm definitely going to remember that the next time I need to do something for someone who is sick.

I must say that I continue to be amazed at the feedback I've received after starting this blog. While it's therapy for me - just tonight I had someone approach me at school to say they enjoyed the blog and that I had no idea how many people were being touched by it. I can't take credit for that - I have to give all the glory to God.

This blog is therapy for me. I'm a words girl - and putting this experience down "on paper" (ha) is good for me. I've warned several of my former teachers not to redline it and check for grammar and punctuation errors - I know it's full of them......but I asked them to show me some grace and just read it for content!

Sending prayers also for the family of a classmate of mine who passed away last night from a heart attack. Awfully young.......life is precious. Every day is a gift. Rest in peace Gary.

So tomorrow I hope to knock out treatment #3 of the scheduled 4 I'm to take of this particular regimen. Treatment days are always full days........blood work followed by doctor's visit and typically a little time to grab lunch and fuel up before the 3 hour chemo session......then the ride back home. The day can be long and exhausting - but any way you look at it - tomorrow gets me one day closer to the finish line and one step closer to being cancer free!

Hugs!

Sonja

Jeremiah 17:14 New International Version (NIV)
[14]*Heal me, Lord, and I will be healed; save me and I will be saved, for you are the one I praise.*

TREATMENT #3 IN THE BOOKS!
August 13, 2017

Well, Friday was my 3rd chemo treatment. That's 3 out of 4 of this FEC Regimen. I have one more left before I start on 8 weekly treatments of Taxol. Another day that I get to make off on my calendar in the ultimate countdown!

The doctor gave me great report on Friday. She said all of my blood work was in line with where it should be and she said that she was very happy with the way I had been able to tolerate the treatments. I had a list of questions to ask her and she answered every one. The first one being about going out in public. Did I need a mask? Was it safe to go or should I stay at home? Her exact words to me were "you cannot live in a bubble." She encouraged me to go when I felt like it.

I asked about school events, being around kids, etc. and she said to just be fanatical about washing my hands. She said obviously, if you find yourself sitting near someone with a cough or who appears to be sick - to definitely move away.....but that it was just fine for me to be out and about when I felt up to it.

We had also noticed what we thought was a "rash" on the back of my head after I had my hair shaved. We took a picture of it to see if it changed or spread. It did not appear to have changed at all. When the doctor took a look at the "rash" - she said it was nothing to worry about - that it wasn't even a rash, but a stork bite/birthmark that would have been there my entire life.......only it wasn't apparent before because my hair always covered it.

The three drugs that I am currently receiving are Fluorourasil-5, Epirubicin and Cytoxin. Some of them are administer in an IV drip, but the Epirubicin must be administered by IV push by the oncology nurse.

- Epirubicin is a vesicant. **A vesicant is a chemical that causes extensive tissue damage and blistering if it escapes from the vein.** The nurse or doctor who gives this drug must be carefully trained. If you notice redness or swelling at the IV site while you are receiving epirubicin, alert your health care professional immediately. (Definition from www.chemocare.com/chemotherapy/drug-info/epirubicin.aspx)

So.......every time I read this it gives me cold chills. This medicine they are injecting in my vein can cause such damage. The nurses have to wear protective clothing (I call it their Haz-Mat suit.)

I was definitely very sleepy during my chemo this time. Must have been at Ativan. I got home that evening and fell asleep on the couch.
After a nice nap on Friday evening and a good nights sleep, I made an appearance at church on Saturday morning. The United Methodist Women's group was meeting to stuff mastectomy comfort pillows.......and they chose this service project in honor of me. How cool is that?
These ladies worked tirelessly sewing and stuffing these pillows. They stuffed over 108 pillows on Saturday morning. They are hoping to donate these pillows to a few different places to be given away to patients who may need them. It was very humbling to know that this group of women wanted to honor me in this way. I'm forever grateful and I know that the 108 recipients that these pillows will end up with

will be very very blessed. I love how God used my situation to inspire these ladies to do something to help others going through cancer treatments. What an awesome God we serve! He can take my "mess" and turn it into a "message" of love and caring from Concord UMC's United Methodist Women. Just doesn't get any better! A very special thank you to each of you who were able to participate in this service project. You ladies Rock!

Saturday was a good day - after going to church, Hunter and I ran a few errands until I got tired. Then I was happy to be home and on the couch again. It was CC's birthday - and while I had hoped to take him out to dinner to celebrate, it just didn't happen. Thankfully, he's old enough to not be terribly disappointed! :-)

Today we went to church, had lunch with friends and visited with my family. I was a bit tired after that and came home and took about a 2.5 hr nap. I feel okay - just a queasy stomach. I honestly think it's caused by the meds I'm taking rather than a side effect of the chemo. But it'll be bedtime soon, and hopefully I will wake up tomorrow feeling better! Blessings!

Sonja

Proverbs 31:25New International Version (NIV)
[25] *She is clothed with strength and dignity; she can laugh at the days to come.*

I KNEW IT HAD TO HAPPEN...
August 16, 2017

Well......things had been going along quite smoothly......all things considered. There had been some small bumps here and there, but nothing major. Funny how all of that can change in an instant.

Today has officially been THE WORST day I've experienced since all this crap started. It's the 5th day after chemo - which has always been the yuckiest day - but not only was it awful because of stomach issues - last night I was pretty sure that I was developing mouth sores........and I was right. Holy crap they are no fun! My tongue feels like it's three times its normal size! The medical term for this is oral mucositis. It's mouth sores caused by chemo (or even radiation). The sores on my tongue definitely make it painful to eat......or talk......or swallow. Fun times!

Obviously, the doctors knew this was a possibility because they had already given me a prescription for Duke's Magic Mouthwash to have on hand if and when this happened. I've been diligently using the Magic Mouthwash all day - swishing it around my mouth allowing it to coat the inside of my mouth and tongue. Fortunately, the Magic Mouthwash doesn't taste awful......so it's not so bad to swish around.

It appears the Fluorouracil chemo that I'm getting is one of several types of chemo that are known to cause mouth sores. Go figure. I've read today that it may help to swish ice chips or water around in my mouth during the first 30 minutes or so of my next treatment. Apparently the cold limits the amount of the drug that reaches your mouth and helps prevent mouth sores. I can promise you I will be doing that at my next treatment.

Between the mouth sores and just feeling awfully weak today - I've spent the majority of the day on the couch or in the bed. Yep - I went BACK to bed today around 1:00 pm because I just felt like crap. No apologies either. Looks like I'll be on a soft/bland/creamy diet.....popsicles, scrambled eggs, milkshakes, mashed potatoes and soup. I pray these mouth sores don't hang around too long......I'm so over them already! Thanks for your continued prayers. I know this is just another "temporary lump" and this, too, shall pass. God continues to see me through each day - no matter how difficult or easy.

Blessings,

Sonja

1 Peter 4:13 The Message (MSG)
[12-13] Friends, when life gets really difficult, don't jump to the conclusion that God isn't on the job. Instead, be glad that you are in the very thick of what Christ experienced. This is a spiritual refining process, with glory just around the corner.

THIS GIRL IS ON FIRE
August 20, 2017

It's been a few days since I've posted here.......this hasn't been my best week, and I have been very, very tired. Taking a shower can make me feel as if I've labored all day. This has definitely been a "resting" week. Lots of couch time........and many mid-morning and afternoon naps. I always worry when I nap so much during the day if I will be able to sleep at night......but so far that has not been an issue....Praise the Lord!

One of the craziest "side effects" that I have experienced from chemo has been a "hot head." Many would argue I've always been hot-headed......but trust me, this is different. At any given time - day or night - my entire head will feel as if it is on fire! The rest of my body will feel completely normal - but my head will not only "feel" as if it's burning from the inside out - it will also be hot to the touch on the outside. One night this week, Hunter walked by me and patted me on the head as he so often does - and he said "mama, your head is really hot." I told him I knew it was - he should feel it from the inside! He asked if I thought I should take my temperature, so we did. Surprisingly enough, my body temperature was normal - but I promise you if I could have just recorded the temperature of my noggin', it would have been at least 140 degrees. I don't know if there is a "name" for this phenomenon - but I do know that it is real. Some refer to it as "head sweats" and others call it "hot flashes in your head." I've had it happen a few times while I was up and around - maybe at the grocery store or running errands, but most often they occur when I'm completely at rest. Who knows?? Just one of the many weird, random side effects of these toxic meds running through my veins.

I admit - every time this happens, this Alicia Keys' song "Girl on Fire" always come to mind.

I guess it was kind of fitting that I didn't physically feel great this week - because I was also a bit sad to see this week come. I've sent my child to school for many years now - but quite honestly, sending him off on his first day of school this year (as a high school freshman, mind you), was more difficult than ALL of the previous years combined. We have never before spent this much uninterrupted time together.......not since I was home on maternity leave 14 years ago. As much as having cancer sucks - having cancer with an awesome kid/cheerleader/sidekick/errand-boy/couch-companion/hammock-buddy by my side since the end of May has been such a blessing to me. Probably not his favorite summer for the record books - but this mama has definitely soaked up EVERY. SINGLE. MINUTE. with him.

He's taken on whatever task that I've asked of him - and many he's taken on without even being asked. He's grown physically taller this summer (and that voice - UGH, don't even talk about that. I'm STILL in denial) - but he has also grown up in ways he could never even imagined. While I detest the reason he's done this growing, I'm beyond blessed to see the wonderful young man that he is blossoming into. While we have made MANY mistakes as parents - he has persevered in spite of all of them. I've thought of this quote many times as I've watched him this summer. This particular quote always spoke to me because while Hunter enjoys watching sports, he's not so competitive when it comes to sports......and that's just fine by me. I can't find who wrote it, but it goes like this: "Your character is more important than how good you are at any sport. Your athleticism is only temporary, but your character, the type of person you are, lasts forever. Be humble. Be compassionate. Be grateful. Be honest and put others first."

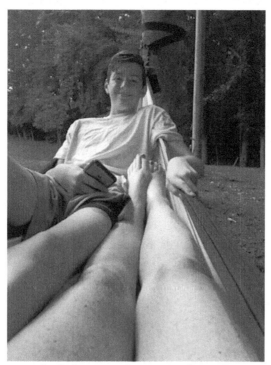
Enjoying a little hammock time with my favorite fella.

He doesn't like the same kind of things that his dad and I like......he dances to the beat of his own drum and he is COMPLETELY comfortable in his own skin (and bright clothes). He is more competitive in the classroom - and for that I am more thankful than you can imagine. I don't have to "parent" him when it comes to his schoolwork. But he is kind......he is compassionate......and he has definitely put me first ALL. SUMMER. LONG. God blessed us immensely with this kid. No, he's far from perfect - he has typical teenage struggles - but he has been a huge blessing to me this summer.

Last week was a trial run - he only had two half days of school. Tomorrow starts the "real deal" - he will be there from 8:00 am - 3:00 pm. I'm happy for him to be able to be back with his friends and classmates and have some "normalcy" back in his life. But I ain't gonna lie......I'm gonna miss him like crazy!

I told several folks at church today that I had definitely felt the prayers of many this week. For on those days when I felt so bad, and didn't know how to pray.......I could feel the prayers of others interceding on my behalf. Thank you to each and every one of you who have lifted my family and me in prayer. We truly covet them and are so grateful for our prayer warriors near and far. Social media isn't "always" a bad thing! I love that my blog allows me to share with friends all over the world - and complete strangers too!

Today has been a long......full......but good day! Didn't feel "great" - but thankful to have felt "good enough" to attend church this morning.......lunch with the family.......an afternoon of rest and Hallmark movies......and I was blessed to serve snacks for the youth group tonight......followed by dinner at my parent's. I'm toast.......but thankful.

Nite!

Sonja

Romans 12:11-13 The Message (MSG)
11-13 Don't burn out; keep yourselves fueled and aflame. Be alert servants of the Master, cheerfully expectant. Don't quit in hard times; pray all the harder. Help needy Christians; be inventive in hospitality.

IT AIN'T ALL ABOUT ME
August 24, 2017

2017 has been an interesting year for us......to say the least. My cancer was diagnosed on May 1, 2017.......stressful enough, right? Then somewhere around mid-June, CC was diagnosed with a herniated disc and was out of work for 6 weeks recovering from that. While he was out during those 6 weeks, he had a recurrence of plantar fasciitis, which he had struggled with since late last year.

**Back story.......this plantar fasciitis started back in late 2016. In March, we had a trip planned to NYC - and he was still struggling with the plantar fasciitis.....and he had a cortisone shot just before we left so he could hopefully walk half way comfortably while we were gone. Eventually, he struggled with it again. Ugh!

In July this year, he had a 2nd cortisone shot and got some temporary relief. He went back to work after his back issues and was able to work for 3 weeks and one afternoon, he said he "felt" something snap in his foot.....and he was again having some awful pain. A trip BACK to the podiatrist determined he had torn his planter fascia. UGH! Bless his heart. So.......he has been out of work 2 weeks.....at home in a boot......just sitting and lying around.....AS BEST AS HE CAN. Those who know me - know that being a couch potato is NOT a problem for me. CC.......not so much. Typically he is ALWAYS doing something right up until bedtime each night. It's just in his DNA. He has struggled immensely just being still! A return visit to the doctor this week and, while his foot is healing, he still has a ways to go. He was given 3 more weeks at home.......in the boot......sitting. If he had an office job, the doctor said he would have allowed him to return to work - but given that his job requires him to be on his feet all day.......climbing ladders and poles.....well, one day back at work would just UNDO the healing that had already taken place.

Gosh - he is gonna kill me for "oversharing" on his behalf. Ya'll know he is the private one. Oh well, it's better to ask forgiveness than permission sometimes.....and this is one of those times! I'll deal with him tomorrow!

While I know this has been a real struggle for him, he has had a much better attitude about it than I ever imagined. I laughed and told him Monday that apparently, the Lord really wanted the two of us to spend A LOT of time together this year.....the only downside was that neither of us were "healthy" enough to spend this time doing anything fun! He's in the recliner......and I'm on the couch!

HOWEVER.......as disappointed as he has been at not being able to work.....we have definitely seen where there were some unexpected advantages to our current situation. I'm NOT a morning person.....He is. The struggle is real! He is up with the chickens.....and lately, I've really done A LOT of power sleeping. Having him here has allowed him to take over my morning carpool duties. He's been able to take the boys to school each day and allowed me to sleep in. The extra rest has truly been appreciated.

Sometimes the blessings of our current situation may not be easy to see in the beginning......but when we take time to "get over ourselves" and see where God is truly showing up...... even in the middle of unfortunate situations, things don't seem so bad at all.

He and I have also had a ton of time to spend together ALONE....which hasn't happened a lot over the past 14 years. We can actually finish a conversation without being interrupted! We've also been able to take care of some piddly things around the house that always seem to get pushed to the back burner for lack of time. We've spent some time watching some of our favorite TV shows.......and having lunch together.....heck, we've even been able to take trips together to the pharmacy to pick up our meds! :-)

Sometimes it really is the small things! Anyway......while neither of us would have "chosen" this......it hasn't been ALL bad.....and we've truly tried to make the most of it!

As for me......this week has been a huge improvement over last week. I've certainly had more energy. I think some of that is truly that I've felt better......and part of it is that I'm slowly (yeah, I said SLOWLY) learning to "just rest." It's still unnerving that I get so tired so quickly......but I've had 3 rounds of chemo......so it makes sense that my body gets a little weaker each time.

Today, I tried to rest up all day so I could attend the High School JV Football game to see my sweet neighbor suit up for her first game. Yes....I said HER first game! She's the only girl on the team.......and while she's a cutie......she's a tough one! I was super thankful to be able to see her run out on that field and attempt an extra point! And it the weather today was PERFECT for football. Not too hot......not too cold!

And yesterday........gosh.....I don't know what was different about yesterday......but FOOD tasted more "normal" than it has since this started! We have been blessed by so many folks bringing food for us during all this......and yesterday, someone brought chicken casserole and pinto beans.

They tasted sooooooo good. I mighta had several helpings of the chicken casserole........and I'm just gonna admit that last night at 9:45, I couldn't stop thinking about how yummy those pinto beans tasted at

dinner......so yeah......I got up and ate a "small" (wink) bowl last night just before bedtime......and I'm not ashamed one bit!
Count your blessings........both big and small!

Now I'd better start working on my "forgiveness" speech.........

Hugs!

Sonja

James 1:2-4 The Message (MSG)

2-4 Consider it a sheer gift, friends, when tests and challenges come at you from all sides. You know that under pressure, your faith-life is forced into the open and shows its true colors. So don't try to get out of anything prematurely. Let it do its work so you become mature and well-developed, not deficient in any way.

POSITIVE PEOPLE
August 28, 2017

I'm elated to report that I have had a great run of good days this past week. Praise God! Counting my blessings........even the small stuff! I did have a headache yesterday afternoon, but a little nap and some migraine medicine after lunch was all I needed to get rid of that pesky thing.

I ventured out to our Personality Festival on Saturday morning. Thankfully we had some cooler weather this weekend.....and being out and about was much more tolerable for me! I ran into sooooo many people there that I hadn't seen in awhile. It's always so encouraging to run into friends, acquaintances and fellow cancer warriors who are so supportive and continue to encourage me in this fight......and I'm still in awe of just how many people say "I love your blog!" God is so good! I have had several people tell me that by sharing what's going on with me on my blog, it allows them to know how to specifically pray for my family and me. While I never considered that as I've written the posts.....there's just another way that God works in the small stuff! An unexpected "joy bomb."

Some days I'm more upbeat and positive than others......but as a whole, I have been very positive through this mess. First of all - The Good Lord has been the source of much of that positive attitude. Literally since the minute the doctor found the lump......I have had a peace about this entire ordeal. He knew I was going to need His help to get through this, and He showed up right away.........by putting this Bible verse in my head as I sat in the waiting room at Durham Diagnostic.......

Deuteronomy 31:8 *"The Lord himself goes before you and will be with you. He will never leave you nor forsake you. Do not be afraid; do not be discouraged."*

And He has continued to go before me.......EVERY......SINGLE.....STEP of the way. God is good.....all the time......all the time......God is good.

My best advise to anyone battling cancer or any other illness or demon......SURROUND YOURSELF WITH POSITIVE PEOPLE! Because you won't FEEL positive every day. But on those days when you wake up at 9 am and just know it's not going to be a good day......then you pick up your phone and find a text of encouragement and a Bible verse sent by one of your POSITIVE PEOPLE......that helps to encourage you to BELIEVE that today is, indeed, going to be a good day. And for goodness sakes, **ELIMINATE the TOXIC people from your life.** You don't need them anyway.......but especially if you are going through a difficult time. Toxic people ALWAYS bring you down - and you don't need ANY of that. You need only positive people and attitudes in your life.

And please know that GOOD DAYS doesn't always mean **GREAT** or the **BEST** days. And it's all about PERSPECTIVE. We have a choice to make each and every day - to decide if today is going to be GOOD or BAD. If we choose to make the most of every day and find even the smallest thing to count a victory that day - it will go in the books as a WIN!

Good days (for me) can be:

- feeling like showering before 6 pm

- not feeling exhausted AFTER I shower

- a day with no doctors' appointments

- catching a morning (or afternoon) nap

- surprise visits to pass the time

- talking on the phone to a friend

- getting emails or texts of encouragement

- someone bringing lunch (or dinner) or taking you out on days you feel up to it!

- feeling good enough to check things off your "to do" list

- someone texting to say "I prayed for you today"

- days with no nausea

And please don't think it's all **unicorns and fairy dust** every day for me! Some days are definitely more challenging than others. Some days, I count it a WIN if I make it from the bed.....to the coffee maker.....and to the couch.......and feel like I've accomplished A LOT. Other days, I have enough energy to make a 2-3 hour trek out of the house.....running errands.....or grocery shopping......or attending church.......whatever it may be. But the most important thing is to CHOOSE to find AT LEAST one good thing about your day and focus on what was good rather than what wasn't so pleasant!

When I think of the positives of my situation - these things quickly come to mind:

- quick showers (no hair to wash, no legs/arms to shave)

- the money I'm saving on shampoo and hair products

- I can take a nap at any time and wake up and not worry how my hair looks! :-) I'm "runway ready" 24/7

- the money I'm saving not being able to get my nails done (yep - that's a no-no when you're going thru chemo)!

- being thankful to JUST be nauseous some days......that's WAYYYY better than hugging the toilet and throwing up!

- being thankful for CHARMIN EXTRA-SOFT MEGA ROLLS!

- being 50 and it being TOTALLY okay to have a PAJAMA day whenever I want to (several of you have visited and found me right here......on the couch......in my PJ's)!

- eating Philly cheese steak sandwiches 3x's in less than a week when things are tasting "normal" because they taste SOOOO......DANG.......GOOOD right now!

- reconnecting with old friends......we really shouldn't let LIFE get in the way.....but we all do! and getting to know many new ones!

- meeting my insurance max-out-of-pocket WAYYYY early this year.....so all my bills are covered at 100%! (that's HUGE)!

Honestly......I could go on with the positives......but I think you get my point!

Staying positive is so much easier with God and positive friends and family on my side. And who am I kidding? I still have a LONG ways to go. I'm sure there will be some tough days ahead......but knowing that I have such positive folks on my team, I know they will cheer me on during those difficult days.

Here's to you finding the positive in all your tomorrows!

Hugs! The verse below says it all........

Be encouraged!

Sonja

Philippians 4:8-9 The Message (MSG)
8-9 Summing it all up, friends, I'd say you'll do best by filling your minds and meditating on things true, noble, reputable, authentic, compelling, gracious—the best, not the worst; the beautiful, not the ugly; things to praise, not things to curse. Put into practice what you learned from me, what you heard and saw and realized. Do that, and God, who makes everything work together, will work you into his most excellent harmonies.

CELEBRATE GOOD TIMES
September 4, 2017

So we have something to celebrate! Friday, September 1st I wrapped up my first regimen of chemo.......finishing the 4th and final infusion of the FEC. Hallelujah! Even though things didn't go as planned......it all worked out in the end. Chemo was scheduled for 12 pm.....but due to computer complications, everything was having to be done by hand and it created a domino effect. I finally got called back and hooked up with my meds just a few minutes before 3 pm. The nurses were working their butts off trying to get everyone taken care of. The infusion waiting room was more crowded than I have ever seen it. Chemo typically takes me 3 hours - so I finally finished up at 6:05 pm. I walked out of the Cancer Center and climbed into the truck with CC and Hunter and off we headed to get some much needed Vitamin Sea in Beaufort, NC.

Satan tried to steal our joy, but we were not allowing it. First the chemo delay.....then I-40 was a mess by the time we got on the road - it was rainy and yucky.....but God was still looking out after us. There had been an earlier tornado and hail storm in Clayton......and had we left at our originally scheduled time, we probably would have been right in the middle of that. So even though the delay seemed like an inconvenience.......God was sparing us from the storm.

It feels great to know that I'm now able to "check off" this FEC regimen from my treatment list. Now we get a few weeks' break and Sept 20th, I start weekly Taxol treatments for a total of 8 weeks. I know I've said this before - but I look at each day as a blessing, as it is getting me one step closer to the finish line......when the BIG celebration will come! Meanwhile, I intend to celebrate every victory whether large or small!

Our sweet friends The Evans Family joined us for the weekend at the beach and we had THE. BEST. TIME. They are soooo much fun, always good for a laugh and JUST. SO. EASY. I've learned over the years that not everyone makes good travel partners. Heck, if we could take on NYC with the Evans, the beach would be a breeze! The Evans are the best!

I had been bummed all summer because I felt like Hunter got cheated out of any fun this summer while he was out of school (compliments of mom "catching the cancer")......and I was so glad that The Evans and their son could join us this weekend.

The boys had a great time paddle boarding - seeing that smile on Hunter's face was worth every bit of effort it took for me to endure the weekend. What a great way to officially close out the summer! And Lordy did we laugh.......George has the quickest wit of anyone I know. You can't be in bad mood and be around George! This weekend was JUST. WHAT. THE. DOCTOR. ORDERED!

The first few days after chemo are always the best ones.....the steroids keep you going. I am so thankful that my treatment schedule and the calendar worked out to make this weekend possible and allow me to participate in some fun. It was difficult watching the boys paddle board from the beach - I really wanted to be out there with them......and while it's medically okay for me to swim.....I am NOT WILLING to take a chance on contracting any bizarre or random infection that may cause any interruption into my treatment schedule.

It hasn't been easy - but I have to remind myself that this is just for a season.....and next summer I should be able to give these boys a lesson or two! :-)

Exhaustion set in on the ride home - but even then, it was a "good" exhaustion - as I was able to sit back and reflect over the wonderful weekend we had. It was worth me being tired as crap tonight - and for sure tomorrow......but I wouldn't change a thing.

You learn to do what you can, when you feel like you can.......and when you need to rest - well, that's what you do. Tomorrow will be my day of rest for sure!

The ocean has always been a place of contentment for me. When I look at the ocean, and watch the waves, and tides.....it's difficult or me to look at all of God's glory and wonder and understand how ANYONE could look at the same ocean as me and not believe there is a God who created all this beauty and majesty.

The beach is wonderful for lots of things. **Relaxing......Recharging.....Recovering.......Reconnecting..... Rejuvenating** and most certainly **Healing**.

At least it is for me. I did a bit of all of these over the past few days. Every night God painted some glorious sunsets for us...and here's wishing each of you a wonderful week. Don't get so caught up in the minutiae of your day that you forget to celebrate the small stuff.

Thank God for your family, your friends, your health.......just be thankful. PERIOD. Blessings to you!

Sonja

Psalm 145:7 New International Version (NIV)
[7] *They celebrate your abundant goodness and joyfully sing of your righteousness.*

SUCK IT UP, BUTTERCUP
September 8, 2017

I've had several conversations with myself over the past few days.......and I've had to remind myself to "Suck it Up Buttercup!" Steroids can be a wonderful thing......and because I take them on chemo days and for four days AFTER chemo....they keep me going......for awhile. Thankfully, they got me through a wonderful Labor Day weekend at the beach with family and friends and I felt FANTASTIC the entire time. Fast forward to Wednesday of this week and BAM.......just like clock work......DFAC (Day Five After Chemo) came crashing in. Wednesday was the absolute WORST day I have encountered during this whole ordeal. I felt like crap ALL. DAY. LONG. Lots of stomach issues.......just plain tired......and the mental gymnastics of trying to make sense of how you can feel so good immediately after chemo......and then the yucky part hits several days later.

Yeah - you would think that one would become accustomed to the routine......but anticipating it and actually enduring it are two different things.

While I enjoy an occasional "pajama day"......having three days in a row this week of feeling like crap has not been easy to handle. I remind myself that my body has endured 4 rounds of some pretty toxic chemo.......and it's okay to NOT feel good - but the reality is it can wear on your nerves pretty quick. I managed to get a shower on Wednesday......but yesterday, I never bothered! I mean, when you don't have to worry about how your hair looks it's not such a big deal! :-)

So when you've spent two entire days on the couch "resting" - it would seem that running to the grocery store to grab something for dinner would NOT be a big deal. Yesterday, I asked CC if he would take me to the grocery store and, of course, he said yes! I got up, got dressed and came out and politely announced that he could stay home - I was sure that I would be okay to make the 3 mile trip to town, grab something for dinner and come back. He insisted on taking me - which kind of annoyed me - but oh well. He dropped me off at the door - and I stopped to grab the disinfecting wipes to wipe down the shopping cart. Once that was taken care of - I was on a mission......to grab the few things I needed as quickly as possible. I figured I should make the trip count - so I planned to get something for dinner for two nights. I was in the store no more than 20 minutes - probably less.......and by the time I reached the check out......I was wringing wet with sweat.......nervous, and feeling like I might just pass out at any moment. Seriously???? How can this be? A little grocery shopping excursion was kicking my ass!

I could not wait to make my way to the car. I literally threw the groceries in the back and settled in the front seat of the car and turned the AC on full blast. I felt like a volcano was erupting inside of me I was so hot. CC immediately asked if I was okay - and all I could do was shake my head "no.".....I knew if I tried to speak, I would burst into tears.

Never fear - the tears came anyway. I had a slight mini-meltdown on the way home......so frustrated that something as trivial as a trip to the grocery store used up every ounce of energy that I had. And mind you - I'd been "resting" for two whole days. What is the logic in that? So I had a few moments of feeling sorry for myself.......and then all I could think about was "Suck it Up, Buttercup." While my situation is not ideal - it is NOT the worst thing in the world either. This quote quickly came to mind....."Don't forget you're human, it's okay to have a meltdown, just don't unpack and live there. Cry it out and then refocus on where you are headed." (Author unknown.)

I guess I'm allowed to have a pity party every now and again......but the most important thing to remember is that I can't UNPACK AND LIVE THERE. Granted - I don't want to even GO there......but I surely can't allow myself to STAY there. Thankfully - crying it out was pretty cathartic......and then it was over......and I got back home, crawled into my bed and just rested.......AGAIN!

Time and God has a way of making us see things more clearly. As I was "resting," I was reminded about all the "good" in my life and that each and every one of us are fighting some sort of battle. For me it's cancer......for others, it may be overeating, or bad relationships, depression, aging parents, financial burdens......the list goes on and on. In the past two weeks, I have learned of 3 more ladies from my hometown being diagnosed with cancer.......and this week I learned of a young 4 year old girl being diagnosed with AML leukemia on Tuesday of this week and started chemo the very next day! I. CANNOT. IMAGINE. what her poor parents are going through......and how do you explain something like this to a 4 year old? This child and her family is having to LIVE in the hospital for the next several months. Their world has been turned upside down! And me......at 50 years old.......was upset just because a trip to the grocery store wore me out. Talk about a reality check!

I didn't sleep well last night.......and that's very unusual......so I slept in extra late this morning.

And so far, I've managed to have a bite to eat......enjoy a cup of coffee......chat with my mom on the phone......work on my blog......enjoy a visit from my dad......received an encouraging text from a friend......and I've decided that no matter what.....today is GOING to be a GOOD day. I'm CHOOSING to focus on the GOOD stuff!

Suck it Up, Buttercup!

Be Awesome today!

Hugs!

Sonja

1 Peter 4:13 The Message (MSG)
[12-13] *Friends, when life gets really difficult, don't jump to the conclusion that God isn't on the job. Instead, be glad that you are in the very thick of what Christ experienced. This is a spiritual refining process, with glory just around the corner.*

BITS AND PIECES
September 14, 2017

Well, it's been awhile since I've posted. That's mostly because on the days I felt like crap lately - I truly didn't even feel like typing. On those days, I hung close to the couch or bed. And on the few days when I felt great - well, guess what - I was busy doing whatever I wanted to do! On the GOOD days - I try to pack in absolutely as much as I can without overdoing it!

The fourth and final FEC treatment kicked my tail......in a big way. This one has been by far the hardest to bounce back from! But I celebrate 3 "good" days in a row......and oh, how I am thankful for them.

Today is a big day.........not for me personally, but for a dear friend and fellow warrior, Renee. This year she has had a double mastectomy, numerous rounds of chemo and TODAY she finishes up her radiation. Hallelujah and Praise the Lord. I know this had been a long, hard road for her......and I am so happy to see her be able to stamp this file as "DONE" and go on about her normal life. I talked with her last night and told her how much of an inspiration she had been to me. We had similar treatment plans, and she has been a WEALTH of knowledge and advice since she had just gone through so much of the same thing. ANYTIME I had a question - she was one of my "go-to" folks. We knew each other BC (before cancer) but we now share this bond of traveling the breast cancer highway and I know that we will share stories for years to come. Her hair is already coming back (and it is soooo soft just like a baby's hair). She has no idea how much inspiration she has given me. I watched her tackle this mess like a BOSS and admired how she has smiled through it all. I have to give kudos to Renee's support team also - she has been blessed (as have I) with folks from all areas of her life cheering her on in this fight. Having a support team is soooo important......and it's truly watching "LOVE IN ACTION." You never really realize how many folks you have on your team until something like this happens. Renee......I hope you get to CELEBRATE BIG tonight! But you and I both know that EVERYDAY is cause for celebration. It's a shame that something like this had to happen to us to TRULY make us realize that EVERY. SINGLE. DAY. is a BEAUTIFUL GIFT FROM GOD! Be thankful ya'll.......even on the bad days......the challenging days......the not so pretty days......JUST. BE. THANKFUL. You may get tired of hearing me say that.......but I will continue to say it because "Cancer Sonja" is on a mission!

I am not thankful for cancer, but I am thankful for what cancer has taught me.

So hopefully the next week will only bring good days! I start the Taxol regimen next Wednesday.......praying I can pack a lot of "good stuff" in between now and then! Trust me - I have some things on my agenda!

CC returned to work this week and has managed very well. While I miss having him here, I know he was sooooo ready to get out of the house and back to work. I hope and pray this doesn't hinder his recovery.

There are many reasons why we love RCS Bulldog Volleyball, but right now, during this season of my life (and in the lives of volleyball parents/grandparents/fans) I am so thankful that these young girls are passionate about raising breast cancer awareness and are having a "Dig Pink" night on Tuesday, October 3rd. They announced this yesterday and are selling t-shirts if anyone is interested! I'm a long-sleeved t-shirt kinda girl! I can't wait to get mine! :-) Hugs to you girls and Carrie for getting this together! You Lady Bulldogs Rock!

Well.....that's the bits and pieces of the past week. I hope you have a wonderful weekend and find something awesome in each day......hmmm....that makes me think about a Gratitude Journal......maybe that's an idea???......be intentional about finding something (or many things) - but AT LEAST ONE good thing about each day. We may have to circle back to this idea!

Hugs!

Sonja

Jeremiah 17:14 MSG
[14] *God, pick up the pieces. Put me back together again. You are my praise!*

VITAMIN SEA THERAPY
September 19, 2017

A good while back, my friend Lisa and I started trying to meet for lunch at least once a week. I joked that lunch with Lisa was good "therapy" because she is such a great listener and always has the best advice. One Sunday at church, our friend Paula heard us talking about our "therapy" lunches and said she wanted to be in on these lunch dates.......and so it began. The three of us made efforts to meet once a week for lunch. We never knew week to week who needed the "therapy" the most! As soon as we were seated at lunch, one of us would always start sharing the dilemma of the day.....whether it was work related or struggles with parenting, aging parents.....the list of dilemmas was endless. These lunches were a safe place to pour our hearts out over the pizza buffet (ya'll know I'm a pizza lover)!

Since my diagnosis in May this year........there were the surgeries, recoveries, and then right into chemo. Then we had summer vacation, and everyone's schedule sorta gets turned upside down. Needless to say.....our "therapy lunches" have been sort of hit and miss this summer. I know I missed those lunch dates - and I'm pretty sure Lisa and Paula did too!

Awhile back, I looked at the calendar and realized there was going to be a bit of a break between my last FEC treatment and the start of my Taxol treatment. I tried to find a weekend during what should be my "good week" to plan a much needed "therapy weekend" with my girls.......and prayed and held my breath that I would, indeed, be feeling good when that weekend rolled around!

God is good.......he answered my prayers and last Thursday evening, Lisa, Paula and I set out for a much needed girls only "therapy weekend" in Beaufort, NC. Vitamin Sea Therapy was just what I needed for sure......but turns out it was what we ALL needed!

What a great weekend of rest, relaxation, reflection, regrouping and recharging. My Papa used to say that the salt water cured everything. I'm pretty sure he was right! I know that there was some mental and emotional "healing" that occurred for me this weekend too! Actually, I think every trip to the beach brings about some "healing." The beach has always been a special place for me......something about sitting and watching the waves come in and out.....time and time again......watching the tides change......all of that is just a wonderful example of God's power and majesty. The same God who created me created the ocean, the tides, the waves.......what an awesome God we serve.

We stayed up late, slept in, enjoyed our morning coffee, ate some delicious food and had NO AGENDA! One afternoon as we walked into Ulta (we intentionally went WITHOUT makeup so we could try some new foundations).......we unknowingly walked right in to an Urban Decay Makeover event at this location. They asked if we'd like makeovers and we quickly said "sure thing." We left that place looking like celebrities! What a wonderful and unexpected treat for all of us! We had so much fun with the make up artists! Check us out #wegotmakeovers #girlslookinggood #canwedothisourselves #shegavemeeyebrowsagain #thoselips

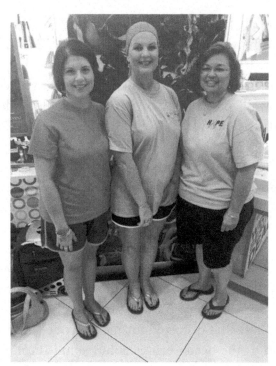

Everyone needs friends they can count on. These girls are real treasures!

So thankful God placed these girls in my life. I'm thinking this may need to be an "annual" outing for us! Our husbands managed so well without us......or was it our kids managed our husbands so well without us? Either way......they survived!

Oh.....if you're in the Beaufort/Morehead City/Atlantic Beach NC area - you simply MUST make a visit to HappyCakes Cupcakery. I know I've mentioned them before, but....Ohhhh myyyy goodness!

Those cupcakes are sinful but soooo good! It's a MUST STOP for my crew every time we come! And for all my local friends - the good news is they are opening a new store in Cary, NC! Everything is made fresh daily. They have different flavors available each day! They really are the best cupcakes I've ever had! Beware the addiction!
http://www.thehappycakescupcakery.com

While it was difficult coming back to "reality".....at least we returned refreshed and renewed. Tomorrow I start my Taxol treatment. It will be once a week for 8 weeks. Praying that my body tolerates the Taxol as well as it has the FEC. I admit it makes me a little nervous.......just like with the first FEC treatment.......my body has never encountered these drugs......I just pray that I don't have any allergic reactions and all goes well. God's got me through this far.......I know He will see me through this next round too!

My devotion for this morning was titled "In Your Delay, Remember God's Faithfulness." The verse was from Psalm 103:2 *"I will bless the Lord and nor forget the glorious things he does for me."* One of the "thought" questions at the end was **"What has God done for you that proves his faithfulness?"**

Gosh.....He's done SO MUCH for me. He has provided me with His peace that TRULY passes all understanding.

I can't even understand just HOW I have been so at peace with this entire Cancer ordeal. That's not ME that's doing it - it's ALL HIM. And I will continue to give HIM all the praise.

By nature I'm a worrier......and I say this NOT to boast.....but literally since the moment the lump was found, I HAVE NOT BEEN CONSUMED WITH WORRY.

It's crazy because I've worried myself sick over lesser things......truly trivial things (when my son didn't get in the school we desired or job changes, you get the picture). But CANCER? That's a biggie!

But I have truly been able to rest in Him.......knowing that He's going to see me through this. And just like He's seeing me through this cancer diagnosis......He will see YOU through whatever storm you are in. Just ask Him! He won't let you down.

If you are looking for a daily devotional, I highly recommend these from Rick Warren. You can have them delivered to your inbox daily. It's a great way to start your day.

http://pastorrick.com/devotional#fullimage7

Blessings for a great week!

Sonja

Jeremiah 5:22 New International Version (NIV)
²² Should you not fear me?" declares the Lord. "Should you not tremble in my presence? I made the sand a boundary for the sea, an everlasting barrier it cannot cross. The waves may roll, but they cannot prevail; they may roar, but they cannot cross it."

TACKLING TAXOL
September 24, 2017

After my wonderful and relaxing weekend at the beach........I came back home recharged and ready to "tackle" my Taxol regimen.

On Tuesday, I was invited to attend a Bible Study at the home of a dear friend and Christian mentor. We had a wonderful time, I met some new friends and we had a great discussion regarding the Proverbs 31 Woman. I'm excited to go back this week as we continue learning about the Women of the Bible. What a wonderful distraction from this nasty cancer and chemo! I was blessed to be able to attend.

I have labs before every infusion (just to make sure all my numbers are where they should be and that it's safe for me to receive the infusion)........and I also saw Dawn, the PA (whom I ADORE). She said everything looked good for the infusion and commended me AGAIN on how well she thought my body had handled the FEC regimen. At every check up with the doctor, they have asked me each time if I've had any shortness of breath. The answer was always no......until after the 4th and final FEC. I told her I'd really noticed that I was short of breath many times since the last treatment. Dawn said that was understandable and made sense because my hemoglobin was a bit low -

but nothing to be alarmed about. Praise the Lord. As long as there is an explanation for it and all is well......I can handle it.

After getting a good report from the PA, we headed up on to the infusion waiting room. No computer problems today - so it wasn't long before they took me back and got me started. I got IV steroids, fluid, Benadryl, and my Taxol. Let me just tell ya that MINUTES after getting that Benadryl - I was feeling really, really sleepy. It was crazy how quickly it took effect.

They advise you drink lots of water/fluids on chemo days.....and I had taken in my share of fluids that morning. I used the bathroom just before going into the infusion room........and literally within the first 10 minutes of getting the actual Taxol - I was DYING to go to the bathroom AGAIN. My nurse was not really happy with me and asked me if I was SURE I couldn't wait any longer. They want to watch you really close the first 10-15 minutes to make sure you don't have any allergic reaction to the chemo. I told her if I didn't go to the bathroom ASAP, I was sure to pee my pants! :-) She reluctantly unplugged the IV pole and sent me on my way......and told me where the red button was in the bathroom if I had any issues. Thankfully - all was well. No need to press any alarms......but golly gee when they are pumping you full of all kinds of fluids, and you're drinking fluids excessively.....trips to the bathroom are mandatory for this chick. I joked that I must have a "pea" size bladder.

Apparently, I got a little loopy kinda quick. My friend Cheryl took me to chemo last week.....and I was really struggling to keep my eyes open and I'm guessing I wasn't communicating too well with her either. She finally said "can you lay that chair back any more?" I responded "yes" and she said "well lay it back and shut your eyes and go to sleep!"

Who wouldda thunk I would be sleeping through my chemo! That must have been a big dose of Benadryl! Yeah....I mighta snored a wee little bit during chemo this week. My apologies to the other patients and the nurses in the infusion rooms! :-)

So.....that's 1 Taxol down......7 to go. Treatment #2 should happen this Wednesday. I've not had any real side effects from the treatment but I have been sooooo very tired. It hits you all of a sudden......like a brick wall. All day Friday I COULD NOT wake up! I just wanted to lay down and sleep. Well, that's pretty much what I did. Saturday was much the same. I got up, ran a quick errand in town and stayed home the rest of the day. I had a few friends here visiting and we were sitting at the dining room table. I finally had to say "sorry to be rude, but I've GOTTA lay down." The exhaustion came on me from out of nowhere. I was sooo upset too because I had plans for Saturday night. These plans had been on my calendar for months. My sweet niece was competing in our local Distinguished Young Woman's pageant Saturday night......and I HAD to be able to attend. I laid down about 3:30 and boy did I do some power sleeping til about 6:00pm. Just in time to get up, get dressed and head to the show. I had prayed that God would give me enough strength to make it through the pageant - and, yet again, He answered my prayers. I mean, how could I not go and support this phenomenal young woman? She's smart, talented, compassionate and oh so witty..... and she fills our lives with so much laughter! She'll always be our "baby girl"....no matter how old she gets! So proud of you Ms. Boom! :-) And so thankful I was able to attend!

Friday I was trying to get some bills paid and was sitting at the dining room table when the doorbell rang. I was expecting someone from the cable company......so imagine my surprise when I looked out the window and saw one of my oldest and dearest friends (who currently lives in Cleveland, OH) standing at my front door.....bearing a huge goody basket in his hands. He was in town visiting his mother and brought me a basket full of all things Cleveland. What an awesome gift. We were able to visit for a few minutes, catch up and have a few laughs. I have never been so shocked and so happy to see someone. While his gift was wonderful......the sweet note he wrote in my card truly touched my heart. He is, indeed, one of my oldest friends......it's kinda cool when you really can't remember a time when you DIDN'T know someone. Our friendship has been around for as long as we can remember. God sent me a wonderful Angel on Friday.......all the way from Cleveland. He knew my heart needed a pick me up.....and who better than Brad to accomplish that task. Never, EVER underestimate just how much even the shortest of visits can mean to someone. Old friends really are the best!

Brad had no idea my son was a Cleveland Cavaliers fan......but I knew right away I was going to have some sticky fingers trying to "borrow" my goodies! He enjoyed going through the goody basket as much as I did. No surprises here when we got ready to go grab some dinner Friday night when he appeared wearing some of my new swag.......but I secretly love that we can share! :-) And FYI - the Bertman's Ballpark Mustard was on point! My only regret is that I didn't think to take a pic while Brad was here. But.....today Pastor Karl talked about our long term memories - and how most often those memories are surrounding relationships. I have a feeling I'll remember seeing his face outside my window for a long time.

Today has been a day of rest and worship......and nothing else. And it felt oh, so good! Rest is good for the soul. Now let's just wait for Wednesday and check off Taxol #2!

Blessings!

Sonja

Proverbs 27:17 The Message (MSG)
17 You use steel to sharpen steel, and one friend sharpens another.

A LITTLE HICCUP
September 28, 2017

I had my 2nd Taxol treatment yesterday. Lab work is always first.....followed by a visit with my doctor, then chemo after that. Lab work was smooth and easy as usual. The port nurses at Duke are on top of their game. Checked that off and went to check in with Ms. Queenie at the Breast Clinic for my doctor's visit. Ms. Queenie ALWAYS calls me by name and has done so since the first day I visited the clinic. I joke that it's her super power - remembering hundreds of folk's names. What a great personal touch! Ms. Queenie is great at her job!

After getting vitals done, etc, I had to answer a questionnaire about any complications, symptoms, etc. I checked that I was experiencing shortness of breath and fatigue. Other than that - no stress, no harm, no foul. Well.....apparently the shortness of breath answer caused me to have to do some exercise yesterday. I was hooked up to the 02 sensor and they had me push the cart around the entire perimeter of the breast cancer clinic. I was doing good on halls 1, 2 & 3 - my sat dropped from 100 - 99 then 98. As I took the last hallway the nurse said "oh my, there it went" and I was like what? My O2 sat had dropped down to 82. Not good she said. She recorded my stats in the computer and I waited to see the doc. I checked out fine but after hearing that I was short of breath she was not quite sure that my 02 sat had dropped to 82. She thought maybe the nurse had entered the wrong number in the wrong place. After conferring with the nurses, they confirmed that, indeed, the 82 number was correct.

Dawn came back in my room with her head down looking at the floor and reluctantly said "well, the numbers weren't wrong......your levels really did dip that far....so you've just bought yourself a ticket for a CT scan today." She was about as disappointed as I was. I asked if this meant that I had to have the CT BEFORE chemo or if chemo would be put off - she said hold on a bit, let me make some calls. She came back and advised me to go to chemo as scheduled and they had scheduled me for a CT at 4:30. Dawn listened to my lungs very thoroughly and said while they sound perfectly clear, she had no choice but to order the CT to rule out any potential blood clots, etc. Not the news I wanted to hear - but you have to know that not every appointment is going to go without incident. The praise was that they could at least do the CT while I was there and I wouldn't have to come back another day. I had to text my sweet caregiver, Pat, who was in the lobby and tell her it looked like our stay was going to be extended and if she had plans, I could call in a 2nd shift. She said nope - she was completely fine and would be there with me til we were done. Gotta love friends like that!

My 2nd Chemo was uneventful thank God. That IV Benadryl is the shizzz though. Lordy, it had me struggling to keep my eyes open within 3 minutes after she pushed that thru my IV. Talk about relaxed. So imagine me trying to have a conversation while already suffering from "chemo brain" on a daily basis......now I'm slurring my syllables and words just evade me after the Benadryl. Good thing Hunter wasn't with me at this appointment. I'm sure there would be video footage of me being a hot mess!

We were finally able to leave Duke around 6:30.......and stopped at Ruby Tuesday's on the way home for a delicious dinner - Pat and I were both starving! It was a long, tiring day but a good day all the same. I was so exhausted when I got home, I headed to bed shortly after getting here and slept like a baby all night long. Long days almost always mean a good nights sleep. And I awoke this morning feeling great.

So the countdown continues. 2 Taxols down......6 to go! I'm making progress and checking things off my calendar. It's crazy to think all this started back mid-April with my annual physical. It's been a quick 6 months for sure. A lot going on and a lot of progress being made.

And those of you that know me know that I am anything BUT a girly girl. Country redneck would be more accurate. My past 2 trips to chemo, it's been hot and I decided what the heck.....I just went in rocking the bald look. After all - it is a cancer center and there are plenty of bald folks roaming around. Pat and I were sitting in a corner in the infusion waiting room chatting while we waited for me to be called back. When we finally got up to leave, a sweet lady stopped me and said "you are a beautiful young lady"....I joked that it must be my hair do......but she and her husband were so kind. I was just blown away. Clearly, it MUST have been the new make-up I purchased on our girls weekend beach trip! :-)

Every day, I am reminded at just how good God has been to me as I've traveled this road. Caring friends, prayer warriors, supportive friends and family, "joy bombs," compliments from complete strangers......the list goes on and on.

Learning I had cancer was NOT good.......but the things I've learned BECAUSE of this cancer has been life changing. Seeing so much good in people, phone calls/texts to make sure I'm doing okay, food, oh the food, and unexpected visitors to bring a smile to my face, folks offering rides to treatment. I've learned that there truly are some awesome people left in this world. I hate that it takes a diagnosis or health issue to truly see that - but I'm thankful that I've seen it just the same.

Now you go be awesome today! And I challenge you to find at least one thing that happened to you today to be grateful for. For me - it was being thankful for friends that sent an unexpected but beautiful bouquet of flowers to cheer me! That makes two deliveries in one week!

So thankful!

Blessings!

Sonja

Deuteronomy 31:6 The Message (MSG)
⁶"*Be strong. Take courage. Don't be intimidated. Don't give them a second thought because God, your God, is striding ahead of you. He's right there with you. He won't let you down; he won't leave you.*"

STINKING COLD
October 1, 2017

Well chemo last week went well.......it was uneventful and I had no complications afterwards.......Praise God! I had told Dawn (the PA) on Wednesday that I had a sore throat and felt like I was trying to catch a cold. Well, no matter how hard I tried to avoid it, "the cold" kept chasing me and finally kicked me in the rear by Friday evening. I was coughing, congested, just plain felt like crap and went to bed with the chickens Friday night. I had recently purchased some DoTerra Oils and I was diffusing oils in my bedroom to try to help me breathe and sleep. I was pulling out all the stops to try to outrun this mess. No such luck.

I woke up Saturday morning feeling like I'd been run over by a truck.......and coughing like someone with tuberculosis! Goodness......I got out of bed, made some coffee and settled in for a day of rest, rest, rest. I nestled into the couch with my coffee, tissues, cough drops, thermometer, blanket and TV remote. I was all set for the day. Thankfully - I never ran a fever! I finally felt up to getting a shower late Saturday afternoon.

Still not feeling great today. I skipped church this morning and just stayed home and rested some more. I didn't want to share my germs with anyone else......and I sure didn't want to risk feeling any worse. Thank goodness there's a new lineup of Fall movies on The Hallmark Channel! And it's been some wonderful, crisp days to sit out on the screened porch for awhile.

No matter how bad you feel - I think fresh air always helps! Hopefully these two days of rest will help me recover pretty quickly. Of course, my biggest fear is that something like this might cause me to have chemo postponed. We surely don't want that.

This Wednesday is shaping up to be a very busy one much like last Wednesday. I'm scheduled for labs, a doctor's visit, echocardiogram and chemo......hopefully in that order. Because of my low O2 saturation levels last week, I had to have that CT scan.

Thankfully, Dawn called me last Thursday afternoon to tell me that the CT scan was normal and showed no indication of any blood clots in my lungs. After getting my results and talking with my medical oncologist, they agreed that since the CT did not give any explanation of the low oxygen sat issue, that another echocardiogram was needed. I had a baseline echocardiogram done before my first round of chemo.......and I'm scheduled to have another one done this Wednesday BEFORE my next treatment.

While I don't want anything to be wrong - I pray that if there is something crazy going on, that the echo will give us some answers. I'm still very short of breath at times - and it's difficult to try to increase your stamina when you plain out feel like crap!

So that's my weekend in a nutshell. It's been a quiet and restful one so I can't complain. I pray that this cold tries to go catch someone else - I surely don't have time for this. I am anxious to check off Taxol #3 on Wednesday - and really don't want anything interfering with me getting my treatment as planned. Here's to a swift recovery!

Oh, and today is a pretty important day. It's my dad's birthday. He turns 80 years young today. Those of you that know him, know that a)he doesn't look 80 and b)he sure as heck doesn't ACT 80! He's a hot mess......but I wouldn't trade him for 10 more just like him.

He's one of the most selfless people I know. He's a people person and if he's your friend - you've got a friend for life. He likes to pick and poke fun.....an eternal "instigator" - but it's all in good fun. My dad has been a fighter - he's shown me time and time again what it takes to look sickness in the face and say "game on" and come out a winner.

He's suffered from Coronary Artery Disease since 1989.....had triple by-pass surgery, a pacemaker, numerous stents and more heart catheterizations than I can remember (although I'm sure if he were here, I could ask him and he would spit out the number in an instant). He's had some setbacks here and there......but his comebacks have far surpassed any of those setbacks.

While we don't always like the cards that life deals us (sometimes we just get a crappy hand, ya know) - he's shown me how to take the hand you were dealt and make the absolute best of it.

Doesn't matter if you were dealt heart disease, diabetes, cancer or asthma.......whatever the illness.......just remember that it doesn't DEFINE you as a person! He never let his heart disease stop him from living.

He may have had to do things a little differently - but he has packed a lotta living in the past 28 years! And I intend to do the same. This stinking cancer is not going to keep me from living and doing the things that I love! If you see this guy around - make sure to wish him a Happy 80th Birthday! Pa, I hope you have a fantastic birthday today! Celebrate BIG!

Oh.......and one more thing......I can't close out this post without mentioning that October is Breast Cancer Awareness Month! Please please......if you (or someone you know) have NEVER had a mammogram, I cannot stress enough just how important it is! Do me a favor - schedule yours this week! Don't put it off. Early detection saves lives!

Have a great week!

Sonja

Psalm 147:3-6 The Message (MSG)
²⁻⁶⧧*God's the one who rebuilds Jerusalem, who regathers Israel's scattered exiles. He heals the heartbroken and bandages their wounds. He counts the stars and assigns each a name. Our Lord is great, with limitless strength; we'll never comprehend what he knows and does. God puts the fallen on their feet again and pushes the wicked into the ditch.*

NO BUENO
October 4, 2017

Today was chemo day! My appointments started at 11:00 am for blood work, 1:00 pm for Echocardiogram, 2:30 for my doctor's appointment and 4:00 pm for chemo. After suffering through this awful cold all weekend......and not REALLY feeling any better until late yesterday afternoon......I was a little concerned that my blood work may not be where it needed to be for them to give me the go ahead for chemo. There's always that chance that something could be "off" and the doctor not let me proceed with chemo.

When I got to my 2:30 appointment with Dawn......she had not received the results from my echocardiogram (even though they had asked for a STAT reading on it......it just hadn't happened). That being the case, she wasn't able to know if my heart could be the cause of my shortness of breath (sometimes chemo can cause the heart to NOT pump as fast as normal and cause breathing/lung issues). Strike one. Secondly, I was STILL short of breath......walking from the parking garage to the clinic, or walking and talking at the same time.....I still get very winded. Cause for concern. Strike two.

Was my cold/respiratory issues in any way related to my shortness of breath? Was it random? Was it totally unrelated? Hard to know. Strike three. Was my body not responding well to the Taxol? (you know that 1% of the population that might not respond well......could that be me)? I think you see where I'm going with this. Today was clearly a strike out where chemo was concerned. Too many unknowns to proceed with Taxol #3. Dawn was probably more disappointed than I was - but I clearly understand WHY she made the call. Too much on the line to make things worse instead of better - especially before she had test results.

Sooooo......this week, I got a ticket to see the pulmonologist.... ASAP......as in before my next scheduled chemo on next Wednesday...... that way, if things were GOOD, we could move on with my weekly Taxol treatments....and should there be any cause for concern, then we would need to re-evaluate my treatment plan and see if we needed to take Taxol off the list of treatment options. I quickly asked if Taxol wasn't going to be an option - would I have OTHER options......and she responded "absolutely."

As always......Kyra in scheduling worked her magic......and I have an appointment with the pulmonologist next Monday afternoon for a pulmonary function test and an appointment to see the doctor. Hopefully that appointment will give us some needed answers and we will know how to proceed.

Was I disappointed? Kinda - but I think God had really prepared me for the fact that chemo MAY not happen today. While I was concerned it may be because of blood results, the root cause was different - but the end result was the same. Taxol #3 put on hold......pending further investigation.

And......as I promised in my very first blog.....I wanted to be able to go back and see how God had blessed me during this entire process......well, here is how he blessed me today.
Just yesterday, I had a visitor who brought me a card and a beautiful floral arrangement. I opened the card after she left. I was surprised to find several vouchers for parking at Duke. I said to my mom that I hated she had spent money on the vouchers - because every time I have

chemo, as soon as they walk me into the infusion room, they ask "did you park in the parking deck today" and when I say "yes," they hand me a parking voucher to comp my parking fees for the day. So I've never had to pay for parking thus far......I've always used the vouchers that they give me at chemo. Well......TODAY......chemo didn't happen. And I didn't get the voucher. Guess what - that gift of parking vouchers yesterday was NOT random. That was God, yet again, **"going before me"** just as he promised in Deuteronomy 31:8.

"The Lord himself goes before you and will be with you: He will never leave you nor forsake you. Do not be afraid; do not be discouraged."

He looked after even the smallest detail of the day......the parking fee. Ya'll......you can't make this stuff up. It's yet another example of just how good our God is and just how intricately He takes care of our EVERY need.

So who can really be upset when God winks at you like that and reminds you that He is still in control.......and I just have to trust Him.

And in happier news......I just have to brag on the awesome folks at my son's school. For several years, the girl's volleyball team has hosted a "Dig Pink" night, where they sell t-shirts and baked goods in an effort to raise money for cancer awareness. Each year the event has gotten more attention and a little larger and last night, they hosted their "Dig Pink" night. These girls, along with some wonderful help from Mrs. Hawkins, their coaches and school staff and volunteers pulled off a phenomenal event. Over the past year - several members of the volleyball team had members of their immediate families diagnosed with breast cancer. The mother of two sisters on the team was diagnosed late last year, one of the team's grandmothers was diagnosed earlier this year and somehow.....they included ME - I have no "direct" connection to the team other than (a) being from a small town and knowing most of their families all my life and (b) the girls being friends of my niece and son. Well - these girls celebrated the 3 of us and others who are fighting or who have fought this nasty disease last night.

It was so awesome to see the gym filled with folks wearing their "Bulldogs for the Cure" t-shirts, pink balloons and banners everywhere........pink roses for those effected by cancer....just a truly awesome night. Even the volleyball they played with was pink and white!

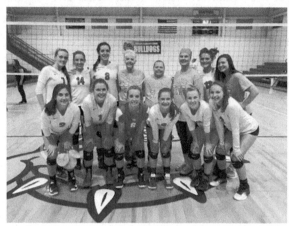

Photo-op with the RCS Varsity Volleyball Team – Dig Pink Night

While being honored by these folks was awesome - what warmed my heart even more was the fact that these young middle and high school girls were "all in" for a cause that had touched them personally. And while these girls make a big impact on the court, the impact they have made on the school and our community and myself is HUGE. At their young ages, using their sport and something they love to bring cancer awareness to others and raise money to for the cause........well, that's making an impact on the community at large. Not only are they great kids and wonderful athletes......they are AWESOME human beings as far as I am concerned.

With such a full heart from last night's event.......it's hard to be too disappointed in my week. I can ride high on the emotions from the "Dig Pink" event for a while. It surely made the news of today much easier to bear.

So girls......if any of you are reading this.....please know that I love ALL of you and I love watching you do your stuff on the court.....and while

I'm proud of you guys claiming your 4th straight conference title........I'm MOST of proud of you for the wonderful human beings that you are.....for the CHARACTER that you display not just when you're on the court, for your actions outside of school and in the community at large. Don't EVER let anyone tell you that you cannot make a difference.......that your voice can't be heard merely because you're YOUNG. Last night was a beautiful example of how each of you helped make a difference. Keep spreading your wings and following your heart and I know that you will continue to do great things.

And that's a wrap. Hope to have more answers by this time next week.

Hugs!

Sonja

Psalm 27:14 New International Version (NIV)
[14] *Wait for the Lord; be strong and take heart and wait for the Lord.*

RE-CALCULATING
October 11, 2017

Well, as you know, Taxol #3 did not happen last week. It was just too risky. Otherwise, I had a good weekend, spent some time at the beach with my favorite guys......went to the NC Seafood Festival (ate WAY too much seafood) and spent A LOT of time resting. (I may or may not have taken some extra-long naps!) The beach is ALWAYS good for THIS soul.

I saw a pulmonary doctor on Monday. They gave me a breathing test and then I met with the doctor. My breathing tests were okay - but showed that I was only inflating my lungs to 80%. There could be many causes. The doctor felt like my shortness of breath and constant coughing could be a form of asthma that is induced by acid reflux. I was being treated for acid reflux way before chemo......but chemo can exacerbate acid reflux, so I had to increase my medicine almost immediately after starting treatment. He prescribed me an inhaler to use morning and night and a rescue inhaler to keep with me for emergencies. My oxygen saturation has not dropped to 80 any more - so that's a good thing. The lowest it got on Monday while I was exercising was 91 and they were okay with that.

The echocardiogram that they did on my heart last week came back normal, which was fantastic news!

So today, I was unsure what my appointment would bring. Labs were great, my visit with Dawn was good and she said that after conferring with my medical oncologist, they felt that it was in my best interest to stop the Taxol and put me on a "sister" drug called Abraxane. They felt some of my respiratory symptoms could be related to the Cremophor base of the Taxol. (Cremophor is a chemical solvent - a derivative of castor oil -- that is used to dissolve some insoluble drugs before they can be injected into the blood stream)......and that, along with the early appearance of neuropathy, a tell-tale Taxol rash on my arms. No matter......the end result was to start me on a new drug. So in my mind I could hear the cool British guy on my GPS saying "Re-Calculating"........just like he does when I miss a turn!

Good news is, they kept me on my schedule - so I was able to get the Abraxane today. No premeds to get with Abraxane.......only compozine for nausea! The new drug looked nothing like the other meds. It looked a lot like skim milk! And it was by far the fastest infusion I've had.....it was done in 30 minutes! No IV Benadryl to make me loopy in 2.3 minutes (which was a good thing, because I'm sure my caregiver today would have snapped a few pics for blackmail purposes)!

So all is well that ends well. I pray that I can tolerate this Abraxane better than I tolerated the Taxol. That being said, I'm thankful that the doctors have an arsenal of "options" for me. And I'm so very thankful to live so close to Duke University's Cancer Center. What an amazing place!

Turns out we just took a little detour......and I'm okay with that. No harm no foul. So today we crossed off treatment #3 of 8. This girl is making progress! :-)

Thank you all for your calls, texts, prayers, cards, etc after last weeks' "delay." I appreciate all the pep talks and encouragement. I was only slightly disappointed. This girl believes in planning and if you write it in your calendar - then it HAS to happen! Well.....not so much with chemo. I'm learning to have the white out handy as we may have to "re-calculate" again!

Blessings & Hugs!

Sonja

Isaiah 48:17 New International Version (NIV)
17 This is what the Lord says—your Redeemer, the Holy One of Israel:"I am the Lord your God, who teaches you what is best for you, who directs you in the way you should go.

GIVING THANKS
October 20, 2017

Well......it's been a whirlwind week and then some! Can't believe it's been almost 10 days since I've posted on my blog......but in this instance - it's a GOOD thing! It appears the Abraxene is agreeing with my body. I've had two doses of it and so far - no side effects other than fatigue. I can handle that! I'm pretty good at "resting!" :-)

The inhalers appear to be helping with my breathing and that nasty cough is still hanging around, but not nearly as bad as it was. All in all - it's been a great week. I got my 4th treatment out of 8 in this round, so I'm happy to report that I'm HALF WAY DONE!

Gosh - that sure does sound good! The Chemo finish line is really in sight now!

Dawn continues to be amazed at my blood work each week - my levels have all been right where they needed to be - no low white counts, platelet issues, etc. and I can only say "Thank you Jesus" for that. I've done so well, in fact, that she told me on Wednesday that for the rest of my treatments, I don't have to come and see her.....I can simply go for my blood work, and if all is well, proceed to the infusion room for chemo.

She did, however, say that I needed to schedule an appointment on my last chemo day because we would have to have a dance party. Dawn loves music - and is quick to whip out her phone and blast a tune or two during my visits.

One day - there was a commotion in the hallway - I heard music playing ("Celebration" by Kool and the Gang). There were lots of cheers and laughter and I had no idea what was going on. When she came in my room, she asked if I heard the music and I said yes. She told me there was a 70 y/o lady in the room next to me who had just completed her chemo treatments like a BOSS - so they had an impromptu dance party/celebration in the hallway! Now that's a doc after my own heart! You've gotta love her!

This has been a crazy busy week. I went back to work for the first time since my first surgery. This is my busy season (Medicare Open Enrollment) and I had prayed that I would be well enough to be able to take care of my customers when the season started.

I'm taking it slowly.....I'm only working 3-4 hours a day.....and that's definitely enough right now. I've come home several days and took a nap. It's exhausting but good. I enjoy seeing my customers (many of which I only see during this time of year) and it feels good to be out and about somewhere other than Duke Cancer Center! :-) I love my customers.....and seeing them and catching up with them has been good for my soul too. God is good......He continues to see me though!

Remember a few weeks ago, I posted about the volleyball team at my son's school (Roxboro Community School) hosting a **"Dig Pink"** night to raise money and awareness for breast cancer? Well, turns out the event raised $3,204.00 and the girls donated the proceeds to the Belk Boutique at Duke Cancer Center to support their self-image program! These girls continue to amaze me.

I am so proud of them and honored to know them! They are kick-ass on the court......but they are some of the most wonderful human beings off the court. I love their sense of community and I love that they have a heart for things bigger than volleyball! They are wonderful young women! I'm also extremely thankful for their coaches (volunteer coaches, I might add)....who have not only taught them the fundamentals of the game......but have been great role models and mentors for these girls. They may NEVER know how much they have affected the lives of these young ladies. Kudos to all of you! Thank you Lord for all of these girls and how they have touched my heart!

I had a late night dinner "date" with my awesome son. I do enjoy spending one-on-one time with him. Thank you Lord for these treasured times! He just completed his driver's education bookwork training today. How can this be?

Difficult to think my kid will get his learner's permit in March! Time sure is flying! And before I can even wrap my head around this learner's permit - he is already talking about colleges!!! That will be here before we know it too! Just knowing that these next years will probably fly by faster than the first fourteen years makes me want to (a) put him in a bubble and (b) soak up every single minute that I can with him.

Time, please slow down!

Well, this girl is about done for this week. It's time to hit the sack and watch some mindless TV! Here's hoping you have a great weekend! Make the most of it - and most importantly, make some memories!

Hugs!

Sonja

Psalm 92:1-3 The Message (MSG)
1-3 What a beautiful thing, God, to give thanks, to sing an anthem to you, the High God! To announce your love each daybreak, sing your faithful presence all through the night, accompanied by dulcimer and harp, the full-bodied music of strings.

REST IS BEST
October 29, 2017

And just like that.......we have checked off chemo #9! Praise the Lord! Wednesday was the first time I just had to report for lab work and chemo (no doctor's appointment in between). It made for a much shorter day!

However, I did miss seeing some of my "people" that I usually run into on chemo days. You sorta become like family with these folks and we enjoy catching up with each other week to week!

Gosh - it's been a wild and crazy week for sure. I had a super busy weekend......Saturday I attended one of the most beautiful weddings I've ever seen. It was an outdoor wedding with a very "rustic" theme. The decor was simply perfect. It was a perfect day for an outdoor wedding! The bride was stunning and it was truly one of the sweetest weddings I've attended. Congrats Mr. & Mrs. Denny! Much love to both of you!

We left the wedding to rush over to my mom's house where we were throwing an 80th birthday party for my dad. Yep - that's right - I said 80! Those that know him will attest to these two things.......1) he doesn't look 80 and 2) he sure as heck doesn't act like he's 80!

We had a wonderful turnout and a fantastic dinner and we all enjoyed celebrating my dad on his milestone birthday! He was surrounded by family and friends .... enjoyed lots of fellowship and probably had a few lies thrown in for good measure!

That was the absolute LONGEST that I've been "on the go" (and I set the record for the most hours I've worn my wig)!!!! I was truly exhausted on Saturday night. But I'd do it all over again - the exhaustion was well worth it for me to be able to attend the wedding and the birthday party of these very special folks!

I've been able to maintain working half days which has been great. It's felt good getting out and about and I do enjoy catching up with my customers. I'm not trying to push it though - trying to keep my work days to 4-5 hours max and sometimes less. It all depends on the day and how I'm feeling. Thankfully - my customers have been very understanding.

Friday was a busy day. A couple of appointments in the am, then off to Durham to meet an old friend and some new ones. You may remember me posting earlier about a former co-worker whose mom was diagnosed with cancer not long after me.

Well, they were in town from Tennessee and New York for a family wedding - so it provided a wonderful opportunity for me to catch up with Allison and meet her mom......my new friend and fellow breast cancer warrior. We had a wonderful lunch (even if the circumstances surrounding WHY we met were less than ideal).

There's something about cancer - it instantly bonds you with complete strangers. But strangers no more! I'm thankful that my blog allowed our lives to intersect - and it was delightful to meet her (as well as Allison's aunt and sister-in-law)! God works in mysterious ways!

I left our lunch date and headed to Duke for my follow-up appointment with my radiation oncology doctor. Now that I'm down to 3 chemo treatments left, it's time to start making plans for the next phase of treatment......Radiation. I admit that while I know it will be easier on my body than chemo - I'm dreading the radiation worse than I did chemo. Chemo was once every 3 weeks then once a week. Radiation will be 30 - that's right THIRTY days which comes out to 5 days a week for 6 weeks. EVERY. SINGLE. DAY. With weekends off, of course.

Just knowing that I HAVE to be there every single day is enough to make you crazy. I know it's all a part of the treatment plan - but knowing that I can't really make any plans for 6 weeks kinda stinks. All of this is subject to change - but assuming I am able to take all 3 of the remaining treatments as scheduled, then the plan is for me to go back to the radiation doctor on November 27th to get marked and scanned and do all things necessary to get me ready to begin radiation the first week of December.

Yeah - that means I'll be doing radiation over Christmas holidays and into January 2018...... BUT I will get a "pass" for Christmas Day and New Years! Even though those days have to be made up!

The blessing in all of this? Well, there are many. I get the week of Thanksgiving off - no chemo - no radiation (if all goes as planned). I am thankful for that.

Thanksgiving has always been a favorite holiday for me - but this year, I think Thanksgiving will have even more meaning and significance. I DEFINITELY have a lot to be thankful for.
Secondly - it's truly a blessing that I am just 45 mins away from Duke Cancer Center where I'll receive my radiation. My friend Miriam, from TN, has to travel 1.5 hrs one way for each of her appointments.

It's really all about perspective. I feel very blessed to live so close to a world-class cancer center. However.......I'm going to put radiation out of my mind until after Thanksgiving........One hurdle at a time.

So my doctor's appointment took longer than anticipated on Friday - and I ended up having a very full day. I was toast by the time I got home. I literally put on my PJ's and crawled into bed even though it was before 6 pm. I was exhausted. Slept decent Friday night and woke up Saturday feeling like total CRAP. Coughing (AGAIN), congested, just felt awful.

I spent the entire day on the couch..... medicating.....trying my best to feel better. I mighta cried a little bit when I realized I just wasn't well enough to go watch my RCS girl's volleyball team play in their 4th round tournament game. I had looked forward to that all week. But it wasn't to be. Praise the Lord our local radio station broadcasted the game, so I was able to hear what was going on. Not as good as being there - but I was thankful for the blessing of being able to keep up with the game from the couch!

And I mighta cried AGAIN when I received a sweet video message yesterday afternoon from the RCS Volleyball team. I love those girls.......they are some kinda special! :-)

I slept til 10 am again today. I guess my body truly was EXHAUSTED. I'm feeling a tad bit better - but nothing to write home about. But, God gave me a wonderful rainy day to spend on the couch and just rest.

And did I mention that Christmas Movies are already on The Hallmark Channel?

So here's to feeling better by tomorrow.........better get back to my movies! :-)

Hugs,

Sonja

Exodus 33:14 New International Version (NIV)
[14] *The Lord replied, "My Presence will go with you, and I will give you rest."*

ROUNDING THIRD AND HEADING HOME
November 9, 2017

So......it's been awhile since I've posted......my apologies.....but between life/exhaustion/work/rest/repeat......well, it just hasn't happened. And this dang time change – whose bright idea was this anyway? I am sooooo not a fan. I literally want to come home, put on my PJ's and do NOTHING!!! Full disclosure: I've done quite a bit of NOTHING over the past few weeks!

Since my last post - I've checked off 2 chemo treatments (#10 and #11)! Hallelujah! I am so close to the chemo finish line!

I can finally see the light at the end of the tunnel. When I went for treatment yesterday - I actually got in and out in record time! Once I get in the infusion room - they get my vitals and give me some Compazine. Then I have to wait 30 minutes for the Compazine to get in my system.

Every other time we've had to wait extra time for the Abraxane to be delivered to the infusion room. I've learned that the Abraxane has to be thawed out before they deliver it.......and even though they know I'm coming for treatment, they don't start thawing it out until they get the okay from the doctor or the charge nurse that my blood work is okay for me to receive treatment. Yesterday everything went like clockwork. The chemo was delivered timely and 30 minutes later we were headed out the door! What a blessing. It was only fair that my shortest day happen yesterday.

It was sort of a balancing act.

The last time my friend Pat took me to treatment - I ended up having to have an emergency CT scan and had to hang around MUCH longer than originally planned. How fitting that Pat took me again yesterday, and we got to record the fastest get away yet!

It's kinda weird to think that next Wednesday should be my last treatment. In some ways - it seems like it has taken FOREVER to get to this point......and then in some ways time seems to have passed faster than I imagined. My very first treatment was on June 28th.....and my last (hopefully) will be next Wednesday November 15th.

Just a few days shy of 5 months since chemo started and a little over 6 months since my first diagnosis. God has been awfully good to me - as well as my family, friends and community. I could NEVER have done this without the support of all of them.

Sunday I celebrated my 51st birthday. It was a pretty low-key day. We went to church and I came home and hung out on the couch ALL day resting up. Then we celebrated with a birthday dinner at the Old Country Club with my family.

I've never been one to dread birthdays or have issues with getting older - but this year.......I was absolutely thrilled to be able to add another candle to my cake! Here's what I posted on my Facebook page in regards to my birthday!

> *Thank you all so very much for the wonderful birthday wishes! I'm always thankful to log another year around the sun......but*

this year definitely more than ever before! For all the drama that social media can create.....Facebook is a wonderful thing on days like today! Getting birthday wishes ALL day from new and old friends and those near and far! I am thankful for each and every one of you and I appreciate you taking time out of your day to send me well wishes! It was a perfect day......church with my fellas......and a wonderful relaxing afternoon spent resting on the couch with full control of the TV remote! 😄 📺 and dinner with the family at Old Country Club! While this has been an unforgettable year in many ways......it has not been all bad. I've learned some very valuable lessons. I have learned to lean on God more than ever before and realized that I'm blessed beyond measure with friends, family, church and community that have walked with me through this challenging year! I've learned that God puts the right folks in your life at just the right times! I've learned to truly 🛑 STOP smell the roses 🌹 and not to sweat the small stuff! This year hasn't been all fairy dust and unicorns 🦄 but there have been many hidden and unexpected blessings even on the worst days! I know that I could not have survived this year without my faith and the good Lord and wonderful Christian friends and family. Of that I am certain. And if any of you reading this don't know Jesus as your personal Lord and Savior.....I beg you to get to know Him! Ask me.....ask a friend....a pastor.....but if you don't know Him, please make it a priority! You will never regret getting to know Him.....but you will regret it if you DONT! Amen! Thanks again for all the birthday wishes! I'm blessed to be here for sure and I'm looking forward to a healthier 2018! Blessings to all of you! 💙💙🙏💙💙

Folks continue to extend kindness to my family in so many ways. That kindness the past few days has come in the way of FOOD! Yesterday I had a scrumptious cake delivered to me and it's been frozen to save for Thanksgiving.

Yeah, I'll be nice and share it with my ENTIRE family for Thanksgiving. Trust me though - it was VERY difficult NOT to cut into that cake yesterday!!! :-)

Then last night I get a text from a neighbor asking if I'd like some chicken soup. With this yucky rainy weather we've been having - that sounded perfect.

Of course I said YES very quickly.......and they made sure to deliver it to me this morning as I made my way to the bus stop! Can't beat that! Then today another neighbor texts and says "when are we going out for dinner to celebrate your birthday?"

I responded "tonight would be GREAT!" and we got picked up promptly and treated to dinner.

Oh......and I can't forget the Krispy Kreme doughnuts! Folks have been soooo good to us - and I am positive that I will never be able to thank them properly.

I just hope they know that we have appreciated every single act of kindness shown to us over the past 6 months.

Whether it was a phone call, prayers, cards, texts, visit, gifts, meals, transportation for me or helping get Hunter here and there......we have been thankful for ALL that's been done for us.

There truly are Angels among us!

So it's my hope that the next post I make will be one CELEBRATING that chemo is complete. Stay tuned because this girl has rounded third and is heading home!

Blessings!

Sonja

Philippians 3:12-16 The Message (MSG)
12-14 I'm not saying that I have this all together, that I have it made. But I am well on my way, reaching out for Christ, who has so wondrously reached out for me. Friends, don't get me wrong: By no means do I count myself an expert in all of this, but I've got my eye on the goal, where God is beckoning us onward—to Jesus. I'm off and running, and I'm not turning back.

15-16 So let's keep focused on that goal, those of us who want everything God has for us. If any of you have something else in mind, something less than total commitment, God will clear your blurred vision—you'll see it yet! Now that we're on the right track, let's stay on it.

JUST PLAIN THANKFUL
November 27, 2017

What a wonderful week it has been. I cannot tell you just how thankful I was NOT to have to show up for a chemotherapy treatment last Wednesday. How awesome was it that I finished up treatment right before the Thanksgiving holiday. That was plenty reason to celebrate and even more reason to stop and be thankful. **Thankful** that chemo was over........thankful that step 2 of my treatment plan was complete........**thankful** for some down time........**thankful** to have a whopping 11 days of rest and relaxation before my next doctor's appointment......**thankful** that I got to spend 5 days at the beach with my family, doing whatever we wanted (and lots of NOTHING)......eating good food........and laughing.......**thankful** that that gosh awful mouth sore FINALLY went away and I could eat without pain.......**thankful** to Black Friday shop ONLINE from the condo in the comfort of my PJ's.......**thankful** to be here.......and extra thankful that God has continued to walk by my side each and every step of the way. Yeah - Thanksgiving has always been special.....but Thanksgiving 2017 made me stop and realize just how much I have to be **THANKFUL** for.

When you pile 9 folks up in a condo for several days.......there's never a dull moment. Lots of picking, joking, watching TV, EATING.....but one of the NECESSITIES of our Thanksgiving trip each year is to get a family photo for mom's Christmas card! Let me tell ya - we have a few photogenic ones in the bunch......but then there's the rest of us. It's easier to get the kids to cooperate than the adults. Some of them won't quit talking long enough to smile......some ALWAYS squint their eyes......some are distracted by what's going on down the beach......you get the picture (pun intended).

Add to that the fact that we have to get our crew together and get out on the beach after we have stalked the beach and we know other folks are out there because yeah - we are that family that just walks up to strangers and says "hey, would you be so kind as to try to do the impossible.....get a decent pic of this wild and crazy bunch." Oh, and it's worth noting that it was cold and rainy on Thanksgiving day....which just made it that much worse. Thank the Lord - there was ONE - do you hear me - ONE decent pic out of the bunch. I'm **THANKFUL** we can say Mission accomplished!

So what do you do when you are just sitting around wasting time until the movie starts? You allow yourself to be a guinea pig! Right after I started chemo and my hair/eyebrows/eyelashes etc started coming out......Hunter went with my mom to town one day and came back with me a set of super sparkly fake lashes! We joked that I would wear them when I went somewhere fancy. I never had long, luscious lashes before chemo.....and I sure as heck had never put on any fake lashes. Well - like a dummy, I sat there and let Hunter and Jalen attempt to put my fake lashes on. Mind you - the lashes were only $1, so they were not high quality lashes to begin with - but it was all in fun and we wanted to see how hot I'd look with these glittery lashes on.

Let's just say that sitting still trying NOT to laugh while those two crazies were all up in my personal space was not the easiest task ever - but somehow we managed. They didn't do too badly considering they'd never put them on anyone else before! Oh well - it was a memory we will never forget.......and I had some sexy looking lashes for a short while......until my eye started watering and I dabbed the corner of my eye with a tissue.....and, then it just started to fall off! I'm **THANKFUL** to have had these long lashes for awhile.......and we had fun doing it too! So today I had my appointment with radiation oncology to get "marked" for my radiation. I can honestly say that today was the most difficult thus far. They had to get my body positioned just right on the CT table first. I had to lay on my back with my hands up beside my head. My head and arms were in these brace-like things and I had to lie perfectly still. They mapped me really good - marking my stomach/chest/side with permanent marker to help them get everything set up for my first treatment. So you know how when someone tells you to be still - you can bet that within 10 minutes you're going to need to scratch your nose, sneeze, etc.

I managed just fine for quite a while.....I even coughed and didn't cover my mouth (no worries, I said "excuse me" right away). They made notes of the position the headrest was in, the table - everything was very precise so that it will be set up exactly that way each time I go back for treatment. I prayed A LOT during the marking and simulation - praying and asking God to please not let me have an itch or have to sneeze or do anything to undo what they had already done. All of a sudden - the cloth that they had placed over me to keep me warm started to aggravate me.....like really bad......and as I lay there KNOWING that I couldn't move - that I just had to endure this - I don't need to tell you that the itching got WORSE.

I kept my eyes closed most of the time - but I opened them then because for about 10 seconds, I was planning my escape. I was all ready feeling guilty for ruining their efforts but I was certain that in the next minute I was going to come up off that table. I prayed again saying Lord, I really hate to do this, but I'm about to bust out of here..... and in the next second, a voice came over the speaker saying "when you are ready, take a deep breath in and hold it for me."

Thank God that she spoke to me right then. She distracted me and forced me to concentrate on taking a deep breath and holding it and I forgot all about the blanket itching me to death. She had me hold my breath a few more times and then politely said, "we are all done." Goodness! I have never been so **THANKFUL** to be able to wiggle in my life! I was probably in there an hour or so today......but the remaining visits should not take nearly as long.

Now I go back next Wednesday for X-rays, etc and I should get the schedule for the rest of my appointments that day. I'm **THANKFUL** there are doctors and docimetrists and technicians who understand the ins and outs of radiology.......they speak a different language......but they get the job done!

Oh......I have to share this story. Friday night we were out eating dinner and I had worn a sweatshirt that night in place of a coat. After we got in the restaurant, I got a little warm, and when I took the sweatshirt off, my hat slid off my head - exposing my peach-fuzz hair do. I didn't think anything of it - I grabbed my hat and quickly put it back on. Later during dinner, a nice gentlemen (who had been seated behind me) stopped by our table on his way out. He said that he just wanted to let me know that 13 years ago, he had been where I was and although it was a long and tough road - he made it through and he knew I would as well. He asked me my name so he could pray for me.

I told him my name, and we talked for a few more minutes. He went on to say that he was a scientist - but he was now a scientist that shared with people how science backs up the Bible.....and he's been busy sharing Jesus with folks over the past 13 years. I commended him on making his cancer count for something.

Before he left, he asked if he could pray for me - and there, right in the middle of Benito's Brick Oven Pizza - this complete stranger prayed over me and prayed for my healing. What a beautiful witness. What a wonderful sight for my son and niece and nephew (and the rest of my family) to witness. God sent a complete stranger to be my Angel that night. I'm **THANKFUL** for that kind man at Benito's who shared his story with me and cared enough to pray for me right there.

Here's hoping each of you have a wonderful week.......and I encourage each of you to stop and take time to find even the smallest things to be

THANKFUL for. Tonight, I'm thankful for a warm house, this fuzzy blanket and a full tummy. And I'm **THANKFUL** to enjoy the rest of this evening at home with my two favorite fellas. What are you thankful for?

Blessings,

Sonja

Isaiah 12:4-5 New Living Translation (NLT)
[4] In that wonderful day you will sing: "Thank the Lord! Praise his name! Tell the nations what he has done. Let them know how mighty he is! [5] Sing to the Lord, for he has done wonderful things. Make known his praise around the world.

AND WE'RE OFF...
December 7, 2017

Well I enjoyed another small break from Duke Cancer Center and Doctor's appointments........I did have my 6 month follow-up with my surgeon last Friday (yeah - it REALLY has been 6+ months since my first surgery).

She was very pleased with my progress and all was well with my visit. She said I will follow-up with her every 6 months for the next 2 years. At the end of my visit - she wished me well and said, "Can I hug you?"

Now you know why I love her so much. She is just a wonderful human being. I'm still thankful God directed me in her path.

On Wednesday of this week I had my "radiation simulation." Can you say LONGEST. DAY. EVER.??? Lying still is not easy for me - and lying still in an awkward and often uncomfortable position is even harder. We had to re-do things on Wednesday because apparently when I coughed once, my body moved ever so slightly (they measure everything in millimeters......so even the tiniest bit off can be a problem).

So.....they let me get up and stretch awhile before corralling me on the table AGAIN. Goodness. I prayed constantly for patience, the ability to stay still......that nothing would itch......you know how it is when you KNOW you can't move - something always happens. One thing I didn't have to worry about was my hair getting in my face! Just a little peach fuzz up there right now! Definitely not long enough to cause a problem.

I left there with my torso and chest looking like some sort of multi-colored road map. They marked and remarked me - I still have no idea what all these marks mean - but I'm thankful there are folks that do! :-)

Because my tumor was in my left breast - I have to do "breath holds" during my radiation. Because the heart is closer to my left breast - they have me hold my breath for 15-20 seconds while they radiate my breast. Holding my breath moves both my heart and lungs out of the field of the treatment. There's always the risk of some residual damage - but the doctor says my heart and lungs move out of the way nicely - so that's a plus for sure. With my earlier pulmonary issues - she wasn't sure if I was going to be able to do the "breath holds" - but my breathing has gotten much better, and it hasn't been a problem in the simulation or in my first round of treatment today.

It took me about an hour today on the table - but the next visits should not be so lengthy. They had to grab a few extra x-rays today as well as get me properly aligned and then my radiation oncologist came in to check me and make sure everything was just right. On my future visits, I'll just go in, get lined up on the table and start treatment. If all goes as planned, I should be finished up by January 22nd. I have a few weeks that I will be going 5 days a week - but with the holidays, I'll have off Christmas Day and New Year's Day and Martin Luther King Day - so that's three weeks I'll only have a 4 day week. So it looks a little better on the calendar than it sounds!

The main thing is **Round #1 is in the books........1 down and 29 to go. I plan to check off #2 tomorrow!** It's amazing to stop and thing just how much has happened over the past 6 months. How far I've come......how blessed I've been throughout this ordeal......and the many wonderful people I've encountered along my path.

One of those wonderful folks is my friend, Miranda. Miranda finished up her treatment last November. She has been a wealth of knowledge for me - and I am so thankful for her. Well, earlier this week, Miranda put this on her Facebook page......

> *Heading to Duke on Friday. I've been having some issues and symptoms, so we are going to do an MRI. Any time a test or a scan is involved, I totally freak out!! It's scary!! You try to stay super busy, so you don't think about it. You try not to think about the worst case scenario, you try not to worry until there's a reason, but it's all IMPOSSIBLE!! So I just ask for your prayers, that it's not a cancer related issue.*

Please say a prayer for Miranda. I completely understand where she's coming from. I hope I'm able to connect with her while she's at Duke tomorrow.....but I know she'd appreciate your prayers. She's been heavy on my heart the past few days. So that's it for now. The countdown is on. Ready to get this show on the road!

Blessings,
Sonja

Joshua 1:9 New International Version (NIV)
[9] "Have I not commanded you? Be strong and courageous. Do not be afraid; do not be discouraged, for the Lord your God will be with you wherever you go."

CHECKING THEM OFF
December 17, 2017

Well it's been 10 days since I last updated my blog. Time flies when you are having fun. Meanwhile....I've made great progress.....I've checked off the first 7 radiation treatments. Wow! Going every day sure does make a difference. The numbers add up quite a bit faster than with chemo (which was either once every 3 weeks or once a week).

The radiation process is quick and painless. The hardest part is being still. I get a total of seven different treatments from various sides and angles. I have some awesome girls working with me each day and they do a phenomenal job. This past Friday was the most difficult day yet.......they had problems getting my left arm aligned properly. It took us about 30 minutes - but FINALLY they got things all worked out. Fortunately, they have taken many pictures to help them know the exact position that I should be in each time. I told them I had some tightness in my left shoulder the night before - it felt as if my muscle was all knotted up. Ironically enough - they said that could definitely be the culprit. My radiation oncology doctor confirmed it and even said that radiation itself could cause the muscles to constrict.

I'm still in awe of all the wonderful folks at Duke Cancer Center. I seriously think the folks in HR have some way of screening the Cancer

Center Employees so that they hire only the cream of the crop. In ALL my trips to Duke I have to say that every time I walk out of that building, I comment on just how wonderful those employees are. They are the sweetest, kindest, most patient and most compassionate folks I've ever met. They work with cancer patients day in and day out and they do it with a smile on their face and a lot of love in their hearts. It starts in the valet parking line......those folks working there are so sweet and helpful and my buddy that parked my car that very first day now yells out to me every morning as he sees me walking in.......then the folks at the information desk are always so welcoming.....as are the folks in the lab, the breast clinic, radiation - you name it. I've truly been blessed by their loving and compassionate personalities. I'm pleased to say that I have NOT had a single unpleasant experience at Duke Cancer Center. Those folks are top notch in my book.

So far I've not had any negative reactions to the radiation. No skin rashes or burns......and for that I'm very thankful.

This past week I had some genetic testing done at the request of my doctor. That was easy enough - they just needed a little blood. Even though I had previously had the BRCA1/BRCA2 testing done in 2010 and was negative for any mutations, they felt that it was important for me to have the genetic testing done again because so much had changed over the past 7 years. The tests are more complex now and because I had previously paid to have the genetic testing, the company did the second testing at no charge. The results came back the same – again, no mutations for the breast cancer gene.

We were fortunate enough to sneak in a long weekend at the beach after my treatment on Friday. Ahhh......the beach makes EVERYTHING better. It was a wonderful time to relax, rest and recharge so I can rock out the rest of these treatments.......and as an added bonus...... the view NEVER gets old!

So tomorrow we will get back to reality.......and checking off more radiation treatments. Let's do this!

Until next time!

Sonja

Psalm 116:7-8 The Message (MSG)
7-8 I said to myself, "Relax and rest. God has showered you with blessings. Soul, you've been rescued from death; eye, you've been rescued from tears; And you, foot, were kept from stumbling."

CATCHING UP
December 26, 2017

I trust that all of you had a wonderful Christmas celebrating Jesus' birthday with family and friends. We sure did. Lots of great food.......family......friends and fellowship......and so many things to be thankful for!

Last Friday (which was my 12th treatment), I noticed some redness for the very first time after my treatment. Fridays are my scheduled days to also see the doctor - and she could also see some pink skin appearing. This was to be expected she said.......and went ahead to prepare me that this week may be worse. She told me if I noticed any bumps or rashes, not to be alarmed - it would be all part of the process.

I was blessed to have a break from radiation on Monday (Christmas Day). Because it was a holiday, I didn't have to go for treatment, which was a great gift in itself! But I was back at it today.

My dad drove me to my appointment this morning, and I successfully completed my 13th treatment. One more checked off the list!

I was so tired this morning during my treatment, I really think I could have slept during my treatment if it hadn't been for the fact that I have to do my breath holds during the process. I guess between all the hustle and bustle of Christmas........trying not to miss ANY thing......I was just exhausted. I came home from radiation today and slept for about 2.5 hours. Gosh - that was some good sleep. I'm nearing the halfway point.....and the doctors had told me to anticipate my fatigue to get worse as time goes on.

I personally think it was a combination of the fatigue from radiation plus just being worn out from all at the festivities of the past few days. No matter - it was great to crash on the couch for a while and get some much needed rest. I was afraid I may not be sleepy tonight at bedtime - but I don't think that's going to be a problem.

Before I started my radiation treatments, the doctor had given me instructions about what types of moisturizing lotions I could use on my skin. They informed that I was to use ONLY things that had been approved by them and to ABSOLUTELY NOT use any lotion containing Vitamins A, C, E or alpha hydroxy acid. The moisturizers they recommended were Lubriderm.......Aquaphor........Eucerin......or Aloe Butter that is available in the Cancer Center Boutique.

I have been using both he Aquaphor and Eucerin. The Aquaphor is very thick jelly (even thicker than Vaseline).......I used it before I started having any redness etc because it took a bit of "umph" to smear it out on my skin. I was a little leery of having to press so hard on my "burned" skin, so the past few times I've used the Eucerin, which is more like a lotion that spreads quite easily. So far - both have worked well and I've not had any issues with using either one.

I'm experiencing some redness from the radiation. It doesn't look like much at first glance, but it's enough to notice.

Can you say "ouch?" I've felt some minimal discomfort from the redness today. My skin feels a little "tight" much like it does when you get a sunburn.

And I have to sing the praises of my 3 radiation therapists......Lauren, Christie and Erin. Those girls are top-notch. They get me in the room and on the table in no time - and have me lined up and ready to go. These girls are on top of their game and do a fantastic job of "dosing" me up each day. I'm so very thankful for these ladies!

So enough about radiation.......let's talk about some fun stuff. Last week, my mom said she wanted to make a 14 layer cake.....but she was going to need some help.

Hunter and I went over last Thursday and helped her make this cake. It was a labor of love for sure.......but I must say it tasted delicious. We may never attempt another one - but I think all enjoyed this one! And yes, we actually ended up with 15 layers. We are overachievers, ya know!

We spent most of Christmas Day eating! It starts off with breakfast at my brothers......he had fresh sausage, ham and scrambled eggs. My mom made 50 - yes FIFTY homemade biscuits for Christmas morning. There were 14 of us there for breakfast that morning......and I can tell you that there was only a very few biscuits left! Later that day, everyone came to my house for chicken salad sandwiches.

I was still stuffed from breakfast but I think everyone else enjoyed his or her sandwiches! And then for dinner we go back to my brother's house for what is always my very favorite meal of the holidays......hamburgers and hot dogs with all the fixings. If anybody in our crew went hungry yesterday - it was their own dang fault!

I pray you had a wonderful Christmas with your family and friends......and friends that are like family. Despite all the yucky cancer stuff - 2017 was still a great year for us. The good stuff far outweighed the bad. God continued to bless us in the midst of my cancer diagnosis. His mercies abound.

So tomorrow I go back to check off #14. Almost to the half-way mark! Please pray that I continue to tolerate the treatments well and that any pain or discomfort I may experience will be minimal.

Here's hoping you have a wonderful week........and close out 2017 like a boss!

Hugs,

Sonja

Titus 3:3-8 New International Version (NIV)
³At one time we too were foolish, disobedient, deceived and enslaved by all kinds of passions and pleasures. We lived in malice and envy, being hated and hating one another. ⁴But when the kindness and love of God our Savior appeared, ⁵he saved us, not because of righteous things we had done, but because of his mercy. He saved us through the washing of rebirth and renewal by the Holy Spirit, ⁶whom he poured out on us generously through Jesus Christ our Savior, ⁷so that, having been justified by his grace, we might become heirs having the hope of eternal life. ⁸This is a trustworthy saying. And I want you to stress these things, so that those who have trusted in God may be careful to devote themselves to doing what is good. These things are excellent and profitable for everyone.

COUNTING 'EM DOWN
January 2, 2017

Happy New Year! I hope everyone had a great time celebrating the New Year.....whatever that looked like for you. For us......well, we celebrated it at home.......snuggled up in our PJ's......catching up on shows we had DVR'ed. It was brutally cold here on Sunday. I've been a hot box my entire life until this year. Chemo changed all that and it seems that I am eternally cold these days.

We ventured out to church Sunday am, then went to town to grab some lunch and met some friends at the theater to see Pitch Perfect 3! It was so dang cold when we left the theater, all I wanted to do was get home and get warm! It was a perfect night for chili beans!

So......the New Year brought good news for me! I got another 3 day weekend - which was wonderful for several reasons. Last Friday I could really see some change in my skin after radiation. There was a really pronounced "burn" area near my collarbone.

The doctor said it was to be expected.......and that I could expect this week to be a bit worse. Ugh - definitely NOT music to my ears. We've been diligent about moisturizing......but some things are inevitable. Having an extra day away from radiation was a blessing.....it gave me another day to heal before getting back at it today and it allowed me, quite simply, another day to REST. And that's EXACTLY what I did. Monday was a pajama day at the Vaughan household. I had NO desire to venture out into the cold so I never left the house.......heck, I didn't leave the couch too many times.

There's been some change in my skin this week – especially the area under my armpit it both red and very gray.

Thank goodness the nurse warned me about that Friday. She said "don't get worried that you may be molding......it's completely normal."

The area near my collarbone is the WORST. It's definitely the most painful.

The best news of this week is that I am now OVER half-way done with my radiation. Today I checked off treatment #17 out of 30. That ONLY leaves 13 to go! Praise God! As you can guess....I've been marking off my progress on the calendar they gave me with my schedule.

Wow it feels good to know that I'm getting soooo close to the finish line.

I experienced some pain for the first time over the weekend. It wasn't unbearable - but painful nonetheless. It's like a sharp, shooting nerve pain sometimes in my breast and sometimes under my arm.

It typically doesn't last very long.....but boy, you sure know it when it's happening. Between the occasional pain and knowing that this week was going to be a little more difficult......I really dreaded going back to radiation today. It wasn't as bad as I anticipated.

I came home and put lots of moisturizing lotion on my burns in an effort to minimize the burning and discomfort.

So this morning as I was getting dressed......I picked up my magnifying mirror to see if, by chance, I may have any eyebrows or eyelashes coming in. Well what do you know??!!! I could see some really really short eyelashes coming out! And yes - the eyebrows appear to be making their re-appearance as well! How bout that!

And just as quickly as I got excited about my eyelashes and eyebrows.......I realized that this probably means the hair on my legs and my underarms may be reappearing too. UGH! I have to say I have enjoyed NOT having to shave!

My mom and I were talking this morning. Here we are in 2018.......and if all goes as planned my radiation will be complete by Jan 23rd. My lump was found at my doctor's appointment on April 17th, 2017.......so I should be finishing up radiation a little over 9 months from the time this shit storm started!

In some ways it seems impossible that so much time has elapsed......but in other ways, it feels like it's been a LONG 9 months.

When I stop and think about the endless blessings that I have received during this time....it becomes overwhelming.

I truly do NOT know how folks go through something like this without faith in God and a COMMUNITY of Christian friends surrounding them and praying them through the good and bad days. I KNOW that folks have prayed me through this......and God has shown up in big and small ways......and it's been my hope that I have given HIM all the glory.

Yes, I've come through the past 9 months with minimal setbacks, side effects, etc. But that's not because I'm any super hero......and it wasn't because I was as fit as a fiddle......I can ONLY give the credit to God. I've definitely learned to lean heavily on HIM and to trust in HIM to meet my needs each day. And He's shown up and showed off......time and time again.

I am thankful that He has given me this platform of my blog to share and this whole experience and hopefully to lift others up.......to encourage those who may be fighting a similar battle......and to just reassure folks that no matter what you are fighting.......you DO NOT have to go it alone.

Many of you have asked what you can do for me at this time. Honestly - your prayers are the absolute best way you can support me right now. Praying that I can get through the next 13 treatments with no complications and minimal discomfort.

I didn't really make any New Year's Resolutions (other than kicking this cancer in the a#@)......but I have made some mental notes of things I want to do this year.

If you've been following my blog since the beginning, you've read where several times over the past 9 months, I've had complete strangers come up to me in a restaurant and ask me if they could bless me and buy my lunch.

I can't tell you how emotional that was for me - and how it was a perfect example of God's amazing love and grace being poured out on me by folks I didn't know and may never see again.

This random act of kindness has really impressed upon me the need to be observant of those around me.

It's my hope that I will be able to pay it forward and do the same thing for other cancer victims that I may encounter. And I'd love to challenge YOU to do the same.

If you see a cancer patient (or anybody for that matter who looks like they may be struggling whether it's health related or finances, relationships, etc).....I encourage you to bless them and pick up their lunch tab. I'm sure you will BOTH be blessed.

Well I'd better hit the sack. I've gotta rest up so I can check another treatment off the list tomorrow!

Wishing you all the best 2018 has to offer!

Sonja

Colossians 1:11-12 The Message (MSG)
$^{9-12}$Be assured that from the first day we heard of you, we haven't stopped praying for you, asking God to give you wise minds and spirits attuned to his will, and so acquire a thorough understanding of the ways in which God works. We pray that you'll live well for the Master, making him proud of you as you work hard in his orchard. As you learn more and more how God works, you will learn how to do your work. We pray that you'll have the strength to stick it out over the long haul—not the grim strength of gritting your teeth but the glory-strength God gives. It is strength that endures the unendurable and spills over into joy, thanking the Father who makes us strong enough to take part in everything bright and beautiful that he has for us.

IS THAT A FINISH LINE IN SIGHT?
January 9, 2018

Why yes, Sonja.......that IS the finish line just around the corner! Hallelujah and Praise be to God. And let me tell ya - I am more than ready to race across that finish line.......but the reality is I may cross it on my hands and knees rather than running or walking it cause goodness gracious this chick is tired.......really tired.

But by golly I intend to get across that finish line one way or another.......sliding, riding, kicking and screaming.......whatever it takes.....by the Grace of God, I'll cross it soon! It ain't got to be pretty........all I want to do is cross it! :-)

So today when my alarm clock went off........for the first time since I started radiation......I really just wanted to cut the alarm off, roll over and go right back to sleep. It took every ounce of energy I had to pull myself out of bed and get a shower......and I stayed in the shower til all the hot water ran out......cause getting out of the shower and getting dressed seemed like just too much of an effort. But I reluctantly pressed on and got myself ready to knock another one off the list.

After today's treatment, I am down to 8.......yes EIGHT.....JUST 8 more treatments. Halleluiah! We crossed this treatment off - but it took awhile.

For the past 2 weeks - I have walked in.......checked in.......sat down......and within minutes they've called me back to do my treatments and I'm in and out in no time. They really are a well-oiled machine over in the Cancer Center. Heck, yesterday, I checked in at 9:22, got called back at 9:24 and I was finished and getting dressed at 9:40 - that's 5 whole minutes BEFORE my actual appointment time of 9:45.

So I've told my friend Pat (who drove me today) to just drop me off at the clinic and run an errand or grab a bite to eat because I'd be in and out faster than we could park. You know what that means right?

Well......it didn't happen. When I got checked in this morning, the board showed that my treatment room was 30 minutes behind schedule. Okay - that's not awful. But my therapist came out and apologized, but said they were having trouble with the machine today and that's what had caused the delay. Truly not anyone's fault - and honestly, the wait wasn't so bad because there's always folks to talk to.

I finally got taken back for my treatment at 11:45 - so it was only a 2 hour delay. But once I got back there - they had me in and out in no time. I was done by noon.

I was so afraid they were going to come out and say that they machine was completely down and I'd have to go home and reschedule. Thank God that wasn't the case. I was happy to take a 2 hour delay.

Side note: (and this is a TRUE story). My friend Pat has taken me to numerous chemo and radiation appointments......and can I tell you that almost EVERY SINGLE TIME - something happens on HER days to prolong our stays. The first time my O2 stats were low and they ordered an emergency CT scan - which we had to wait for......and got home after dinner! The next time it took FOREVER for my chemo to thaw out that day........and today, the Green Machine was acting up. I can't tell you how much I hated texting her to say "yet again......there's been a delay."......it's really become quite comical at this point! (Well - maybe not to her!) :-)

But in true Pat fashion - she just smiled and said "the Lord evidently wanted us to spend a little more time together today!" And she drops me back off at home and says "let me know when you need me again!" Yes......I've been blessed!

As the old saying goes, I'm "in the short rows" now. And not a minute too soon. I'm definitely ready to NOT have my calendar planned out for me! I may not know how to act when I'm not headed to Durham every day.

The doctor told me on Friday that the next two weeks would be the worst. This week I continue getting the same treatment as always but the last 5 days I will get a "boost" and they will target the tumor bed during those 5 treatments. My skin has definitely become more sensitive as the "burning" has gotten worse.

The one area near my collarbone is still the WORST and the back of my shoulder is quite tender. I've encountered some swelling over the past week and the doctor said that was to be expected and she has me taking ibuprofen 3x's a day to help with the swelling and the pain.

The last few days there's been a shooting pain in my breast. It comes and goes - but it is quite uncomfortable and extremely annoying. Itching is the worst at night - I guess when I get all snuggled up under the covers, I get "just warm enough" for the itching to begin. I've taken a Benadryl the last few nights so I wouldn't wake up clawing myself. You know how when you get a sunburn and your skin feels really really tight......that's how this feels too.

The area near my collarbone is by far the worst and most painful......... But all in all........the pain, discomfort, the traveling, the early mornings, the burning, the itching......it has not been unbearable. And when I find myself wanting to be a little whiny - I have to stop and remind myself that ALL of the pain and discomfort I've experienced - if I bottled it all up together would be but a drop in the bucket to the pain that Jesus endured on The Cross. THAT - was suffering.

So if Jesus could endure The Cross for me (and you) - then I can definitely endure this with His help........as it pales by comparison.

I've often said that I considered it quite an honor that God allowed me to be able to participate with HIM in the miracle of childbirth. And we all know that a typical pregnancy lasts 9 months.

When you think about ALL the things that must happen to create a living breathing child inside your womb - it's nothing short of a miracle.

After I was diagnosed with cancer, I remember telling some friends that I felt like God was going to allow me to participate in yet another miracle with Him.......that he would heal me of this cancer and allow me to use my story to truly glorify Him.

Today, as I sat and did the math (and yes, I checked my numbers several times because we ALL know that math is not my strong suit).......this whole mess started in April 17, 2017........and if all goes as planned, I should finish up treatment on Jan 22, 2018. You do the math behind me! :-)

That's a little over 9 months since this whole mess started. **#truth** I just chuckled to myself.

Isn't that just like God!?

We sang this song in church Sunday........WOW.....did it speak directly to me. I love it! Hope you enjoy!

Gracefully Broken by Matt Redman

https://www.youtube.com/watch?v=IJNR0lxbIP4

Love and hugs,

Sonja

Hebrews 12:1-3 The Message (MSG)
¹⁻³*Do you see what this means—all these pioneers who blazed the way, all these veterans cheering us on? It means we'd better get on with it. Strip down, start running—and never quit! No extra spiritual fat, no parasitic sins. Keep your eyes on Jesus, who both began and finished this race we're in. Study how he did it. Because he never lost sight of where he was headed—that exhilarating finish in and with God—he could put up with anything along the way: Cross, shame, whatever. And now he's there, in the place of honor, right alongside God. When you find yourselves flagging in your faith, go over that story again, item by item, that long litany of hostility he plowed through. That will shoot adrenaline into your souls!*

SOOOOO CLOSE
January 16, 2018

Well ya'll, I'm getting soooo close to being done! I finished up my scheduled radiation treatments last Friday. I was set for a total of 25 and we checked #25 off on Friday. My appointment was a little longer than normal because immediately after my treatment Friday, they began marking me up and getting the machines set up for the next series of 5 "boost" treatments......and the doctor had to come in and make sure everything was set up as it should be. These 5 treatments will specifically target the tumor bed. My incision from the lumpectomy surgery is under my left arm pit. The machine is set up very close to my incision site - and they radiate me for about 20 seconds each day and that's it.

Last week was by far the hardest yet. Not in terms of pain or anything - just getting up and getting going. The fatigue showed up big time......and even though you know to expect it.......I don't think you are ever quite prepared for how quickly it comes on at times.

Like one minute you feel great and full of energy and 10 minutes later, you've hit a brick wall and getting off of the couch to get a snack seems like too much of an effort. Craziness!

With Monday being a holiday - my son was out of school and I had the day off from radiation.......so we decided it was a perfect weekend to head down to the beach. Who cares if it was freezing cold.

The beach makes everything better. My mom and dad were able to join us - and we had a great time just hanging out, watching TV, eating good, watching for horses on the island, and lounging in our PJ's.........it was just what the doctor ordered.

And speaking of mom and dad.......let me just say that I can never thank them enough for ALL the help and support they have offered me since all this mess began.

Whether it was moral support.......or accompanying me to doctors' appointments........or chemo........or driving me to radiation.........or making sure Hunter had transportation to school or dental appointments........or picking me up a loaf of bread so I'd be prepared for Snowmageddon (not just ANY bread, it HAS to be the BEST bread in town from IGA!)......they have gone above and beyond to support me and I will be forever grateful for all they have done. Honestly, I hit the jackpot when it comes to parents (and Hunter, Jalen and Haden hit the MegaMillions in the grandparent category for sure). My parents are two of the most giving and selfless folks that I know......and I'm glad that God chose them to be mine.

Today was my first "boost" and it was quick and painless. Truthfully, it takes me longer to change from my clothes into the hospital gown than the treatment takes! All I have to do is lay there......completely still.......but this time I don't have to do any breath holds so it's super quick and easy. So I've got 1 down and 4 to go. And yeah - they are calling for lots of snow tonight......so I'm praying I can get #2 in the books tomorrow. I'll have to call them in the morning to see if they are operating on regular schedule or not.....or if I need to come in at a later time. I've all ready advised my brother that I'll need him to get me over there if the snow comes.....so we're all set to get there provided we can do it safely. I'm too close to the end now to let a little snow stand in the way!

I also had a follow-up appointment with the pulmonary doctor this afternoon. My latest pulmonary function test was completely normal.......so he's taking me off of my daily inhaler. While it's difficult to know if the asthma was brought on by an allergic reaction to the chemo Taxol.......or from me being anemic........I'm just glad it's gone. He wants me to continue to carry my rescue inhaler as a precaution. He said cold weather can definitely induce breathing problems (and baby, it's definitely cold outside)!

I will follow up with him in 6 months just to be sure I don't have any pulmonary issues after completing radiation and he will probably repeat my pulmonary function test at that time. Hooray for a great report!

So here's how things looked once I wrapped up my 25 treatments. The collar bone area took the worst beating......but it's healing up a bit. She prescribed me some silvadene cream to apply to that area. Please know I don't talk about these burns, or anything cancer-related, to be boastful in any way. As I mentioned in my very first blog entry - my goal was to be as open and honest and authentic as I could. Not to pat myself on the back - but to encourage others who may be going through something similar. To see that it's DOABLE.....it may not be pretty - and it may not be fun - but in the end, it is DOABLE.

The center of my chest is by far the place that itches the most. It's starting to peel like a sunburn would.....so hopefully that's starting to heal as well. I'm expecting the area under my arm to get a little more tender since these last boosts focus directly on that area......but so far so good.

My hair has really grown A LOT over the past two weeks. Let's just say that it's a tad bit lighter than I remembered! :-) That's okay - I'll take it. And somehow.....somewhere in the middle of all of this.......hairy legs happened! Ugh......seriously? I have NOT missed shaving my legs lemme tell ya! I was sooo sad to see THAT hair growing back!

Well......it's time to call it a night. Hang on a few more days........I'm so close I can almost taste it! :-)

Blessings!

Sonja

2 Corinthians 4:16-17 New Living Translation (NLT)
¹⁶*That is why we never give up. Though our bodies are dying, our spirits are being renewed every day.* ¹⁷*For our present troubles are small and won't last very long. Yet they produce for us a glory that vastly outweighs them and will last forever!*

REALLY NOW?
January 21, 2018

Ever feel like some days or weeks that the deck has been stacked against ya? Satan tried every way he could this past week to steal my joy. It started last weekend with the weather reports calling for snow last Wednesday.........really? Right in the middle of my home stretch? I can promise you that being 26 treatments in - I wanted NOTHING to interfere with me making it to my next 4 appointments and getting those things DONE. Add to that that I'm TOTALLY not a fan of winter (I'll take the 70's and flip flops ANY day).....well, this chick was NOT a happy camper.

Thankfully - the snow didn't start here until 5:30ish that morning. My husband HAS to work no matter the weather.......and fortunately for me - my brother can't really work when it snows - so he was at home and offered to get me to Duke. The roads were not great - thank God he had 4-wheel drive and I'm even more thankful that, unlike me - he isn't afraid of driving in that mess. We made it to and from Duke without incident - but saw a lot of cars in the ditch and accidents along the way. Treatment #27 - DONE!

After I got home - it continued to snow. It snowed.......and snowed......and snowed......we had 12+ hours of snowfall here in little

Siberia (aka Roxboro) and well over 12 inches of snow! I admit it was absolutely beautiful coming down - and it creates a beautiful backdrop for all of God's creation.......but golly gee - all this snow was surely going to make getting back to Duke on Thursday a royal pain in the butt.

Thankfully......Kippy said he would be glad to take me again on Thursday. Because of the inclement weather, Radiation Oncology was not opening until 10:00 am on Thursday. We made it back to Duke and I was in and out of my appointment in no time and headed back home. Treatment #28 - DONE!

Friday my dad offered to take me to treatment. They were opening at 9am Friday morning - so I was still able to go at my regular 9:45am time. I checked in, sat down - well, I think my butt actually hit the seat of the chair and almost immediately I was called back for treatment. Those girls were rocking us in and out of The Green Room on Friday! Treatment #29 was IN THE BOOKS.

I know this is going to sound crazy to most of you - but I'm going to miss my girls in The Green Room. When you spend 30 days with your radiation therapists - you really get to know them and they become like part of your family.

They have been soooo awesome to work with and have made this whole experience much more bearable. They are 3 of the sweetest girls I've ever met. So I gave them fair warning on Friday that they had all weekend to wrap their brains about the fact that I would be breaking up with them on Monday! Those girls NEVER know what I'm gonna say! Monday would be my 30th and final treatment - and I just wanted them to prepare themselves! :-)

Every Friday after treatment, I see my radiation oncologist. This would be my last visit with her for a while as well. She came in the room with a certificate in her hand - kinda cool that I get a certificate for completing radiation!

So.....as she sat down to talk to me - she informed me that it turns out that Monday WON'T be my final radiation treatment. WHAT??? She had decided to give me one additional "boost" treatment in order to get the total dose of radiation she desired for me........so while she had brought me a certificate of completion......upon more careful inspection, the date she had entered on the certificate was, indeed, Tuesday, January 23rd!

Well......what's one more day? And honestly - I have to be in Durham Tuesday am anyway for Hunter's orthodontist appointment - so it wasn't going to be a huge imposition. Honestly......if she feels that one more dose was needed to keep that nasty cancer from coming back - by ALL MEANS, let's do it. The stinking treatment only lasts 20 seconds so it's really not a big deal.

We discussed my follow up appointments........I won't see her again until the fall.....but she said that I won't get much of a break from doctors appointments for the rest of this year....I'll be in and out between return visits with the medical oncologist, my surgeon and the radiation oncologist......and follow up mammograms, etc.

She laughed and said I'd get a break from so many appointments NEXT year and should only see each of them once a year if all goes well.

So between the snow......the yucky roads......transportation worries......and an unexpected extra radiation treatment.......Satan tried to take up some real estate in my life......but we had no time for that. As always......God provided.....Just what I needed......Just in time.....and brought me JOY!

Thankful that even in the midst of all of this.....God continues to reassure me that HE is in control......that HE has me.......and that He will see me through.

We're ALMOST there.........

Hugs!

Sonja

Psalm 94:19 New International Version (NIV)

[19] When anxiety was great within me, your consolation brought me joy.

AND WE'RE DONE!
January 23, 2018

And that's a WRAP! Yep.......today I walked out of Duke Cancer Center Radiation Oncology Department with a flood of emotions as I completed my 31st and final treatment. What an incredible feeling. I'm not really sure I'm going to know what to do with myself now that I have an entire week of no doctor's appointments/treatments, etc.

I stopped to take a pic of the EXIT just before I walked out of there this morning. What a welcome sight!

Walking into my treatment this morning - I was so happy and eager to get this, the FINAL one in the books. The girls got me adjusted on the table and as they walked out the door to go get ready for my treatment - it really hit me that this was IT.......this long awaited final treatment was finally going to happen......and then the tears just came......and came. I think I became overwhelmed at just everything that had transpired over the past nine months......the good and the bad........and the tears proved to be very cathartic and probably long overdue.

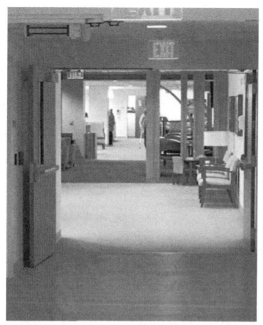

The final exit......a long time coming.

Yeah - I know this is gonna sound crazy........but I'm really going to miss seeing my 3 radiation therapists. I'm pretty biased, but I think I had the absolute BEST therapists on the planet. Christie, Erin and Lauren were amazing and took such great care of me.

God definitely gave each of them a heart for serving and caring for others and I'm thankful that I got to know them......but I hope the next time I see them it's at the mall or somewhere FUN! Margaritas maybe??!! I couldn't have done it without them cheering me on!

And the parking attendant, Ahmed.....he has been the absolute BEST.

From the first day of radiation when I wasn't sure where to park or what to do......he explained the drill to me and what I needed to do......and EVERY MORNING SINCE he has yelled "Good Morning" to me from across the way.
I don't care if I parked in the deck, did valet or got dropped off - this fella saw me each and every day and always had a big smile and well wishes for the day.

Now THAT'S going above and beyond! He even put his chap stick on so he was picture ready!

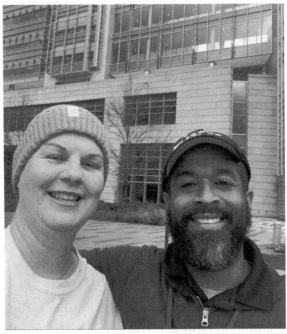

This guy right here greeted me EVERY SINGLE DAY. He's amazing!

So guess what?? This chick ain't setting an alarm for tomorrow!! I have NO WHERE that I have to be.

What a blessing! Granted......the fatigue is still hanging around like a bad cold......and it's not going anywhere anytime soon so I'm told.

But that's okay. I'll just plan to "watch Netflix and chill" for a while.

I follow up with my medical oncologist next week......to discuss immunotherapy and next steps. My Duke My Chart is already full of return appointments.....with the surgeon, for my mammogram, follow-ups with medical and radiation oncologists, labs, etc.

So I'm far from being DONE - but the 3 biggest hurdles are behind me - surgery, chemo and radiation! That's definitely cause for a celebration.

Kyra and Byron - I see some mango margaritas in our future!

And let me just say again how thankful I am that I live so close to such a world renowned facility like Duke Cancer Center. I'm fortunate to only have to travel 32 miles to get there......I've met so many folks from near and far who travel many miles and hours to get top notch care from some of the best physicians and people on the planet.

I'm definitely thankful to be just a short drive away. I honestly cannot say enough just how awesome everyone I've encountered has been. They are definitely top notch over there!

Now I'm off to enjoy an entire week of NO APPOINTMENTS!

Halleluiah!

> *Thank you Lord for seeing me through these past nine months. For never once forsaking me........for being available day or night when I cried out to you......for showing me your Mercy and Grace time and time again.......for holding me up when I was too weak to stand on my own.......and sending me angels in so many forms........I cannot take credit for making it to this point. For that - I give you all the glory, honor and praise......and I humbly thank you for all the blessings you have shown me (both big and small) along the way. Amen.*

Blessings,

Sonja

(So I really liked both of these versions of Acts 20:24.......and I couldn't share just one!)

Acts 20:24 New Living Translation (NLT)
[24] *But my life is worth nothing to me unless I use it for finishing the work assigned me by the Lord Jesus—the work of telling others the Good News about the wonderful grace of God.*

Acts 20:24 The Message (MSG)
[22-24] *"But there is another urgency before me now. I feel compelled to go to Jerusalem. I'm completely in the dark about what will happen when I get there. I do know that it won't be any picnic, for the Holy Spirit has let me know repeatedly and clearly that there are hard times and imprisonment ahead. But that matters little. What matters most to me is to finish what God started: the job the Master Jesus gave me of letting everyone I meet know all about this incredibly extravagant generosity of God.*

FINDING MY NEW NORMAL
January 31, 2018

It's now been exactly one week since I completed my last radiation treatment. And what a wonderful week it's been. I really can't describe just how awesome it's been to have NOTHING on my calendar. No labs......no doctor's appointments......no treatments...... NOTHING! It's quite a welcome change!

The fatigue is still a big issue - and Saturday I took the liberty of having a "pajama day." I had the most relaxing day at home doing NOTHING and it was wonderful. This week, however, I'm trying to MAKE myself get up and do SOMETHING each day. Even if it's only for a few hours. Sometimes - just getting up and getting moving helps.

Call me crazy (you won't be the first).....but last week, for the first time since my cancer diagnosis......I truly experienced a little fear. How crazy is it that this fear only showed up AFTER the chaos of the past nine months.......AFTER all the hard stuff was over.

But a few days after completing radiation - I had this realization that there had been a HUGE sense of security during all my chemo and radiation treatments. I was constantly at the hospital, having blood work, getting chemo or radiation, and X-rays, and weekly visits with the doctor......but NOW......all of that is over. I mean, I'll still have sporadic visits with the doctors but nothing like before. Being at the hospital so much, there was this enormous sense of security regarding my health - because they were constantly checking me and looking out for me.

Now.....well, that FEAR crept in big time last week. I remember having a conversation with myself (don't judge) saying "here is where you find out just how big your faith is." I admit that I have had the utmost faith in my doctors, nurses, therapists, etc. from the beginning. Faith that they were going to do the absolute best they could in efforts to rid my body of this cancer. I've also had faith that God was going to see me through this - whatever that looked like.....but that FEAR kept creeping in. Was I really going to be able to trust and believe that I had been healed? Was I going to have the confidence to move forward with my life and not let this fear paralyze me?

I messaged my friend Miranda saying "while I'm happy to be done with treatment, there was always this sense of security being at the hospital every single day." She responded back confirming that what I was feeling was completely normal.......and while it does get better, it takes awhile. Okay - so at least there was some validity to what I was feeling......and obviously others have experienced this same fear as well.

So......let me set the stage for what happened next.

Several weeks ago, my friend Lisa felt led to start a Bible Study in her home. We were going to meet on Friday nights. The first week she held the class, I was out of town, so I was unable to go. The next week, we got hit by a small blizzard in the middle of the week.....and because there was still snow and ice hanging around, she decided it was best to cancel that Friday. Here is what she posted about cancelling that night (January 19th was the actual date).

> *Bible study at my home is canceled for tonight. While the roads are clear, Westover and my driveway are still pretty icy. I am most concerned about someone slipping and falling while getting*

from the road into the house. We will resume next Friday at 6:30 p.m. Come and enjoy! Our topic will still be "Walking from fear into faith." It will be a great time! Hope to see you!

So.....last week we were able to meet on Friday night at her home. Our topic was "Walking from fear into faith"......the study she had prepared the week prior before the Snowpocalypse. We discussed that fear is real. And fear is designed by God to alert us to danger......and it's not realistic to think we can live without fear at times.

Psalm 56:3-4: *"But when I am afraid, I will put my trust in you. I praise God for what he has promised. I trust in God, so why should I be afraid? What can mere mortals do to me?"*

Hebrews 11:1 *"Now Faith is confidence in what we hope for and assurance about what we do not see."*

So was my faith, indeed, bigger than my fear? As I sat there Friday night - I wasn't sure why anybody else had come, because I was CONFIDENT that God intended this message JUST FOR ME.

Isn't it cool to sit back and look at how God works? You see - the Friday before (the original date we were to discuss this topic) I still had two radiation treatments left.

I had not yet felt this fear creep in. God's timing is always perfect. And although Lisa had prepared this study a week prior - God knew that these fears were going to creep in for me last week. He knew just when I needed to hear this!

Once again - I got cold chills.

We also discussed these 4 Truths:

#1 - God Loves us (as shown in John 3:16, John 16:27 and Romans 5:5)

#2 - God knows what is going on in our lives (Matthew 6:31-32, Psalms 139:1-10)

$3 - God can do something about it (Genesis 18:14, Luke 1:37)

#4 - You can trust His goodness in whatever He chooses to do (Proverbs 3:5, Psalms 119:68)

For obvious reasons - Truth #2 really stood out to me. God knows what's going on in my life (just like He knows what's going on in yours). He knows my fears - and He knew those fears were going to creep in......and HE knew I needed to hear this study on that very topic on this exact night!

Before we wrapped up our study Friday night, we listened to this song "Trust in You" by Laura Daigle.

I've heard this song many, many times......but on this particular night, the words resonated with me like never before. The verse at the 1:17 minute mark really spoke to me

> *Truth is, You know what tomorrow brings/There's not a day ahead You have not seen/So let all things be my life and breath I want what You want Lord and nothing less*

https://www.youtube.com/watch?v=n_aVFVveJNs

Yet again......God showed up and showed off. On so many levels. I'm so thankful for my friend Lisa - and for her stepping out in faith to start this Bible Study in her home (and trust me, she had MANY fears about doing this). Because her faith was bigger than her fear - she was obedient to what God had laid on her heart to do........and God used her and her Bible Study to speak directly to ME about MY faith and MY fear. How awesome is that??!!!

I love that God continues to remind me to "keep your eyes on ME!"

Be Blessed!

Sonja

Psalm 139:1-10 New International Version (NIV)
^{1}You have searched me, Lord, and you know me. ^{2}You know when I sit and when I rise; you perceive my thoughts from afar. ^{3}You discern my going out and my lying down; you are familiar with all my ways. ^{4}Before a word is on my tongue you, Lord, know it completely. ^{5}You hem me in behind and before, and you lay your hand upon me. ^{6}Such knowledge is too wonderful for me, too lofty for me to attain. ^{7}Where can I go from your Spirit? Where can I flee from your presence? ^{8}If I go up to the heavens, you are there; if I make my bed in the depths, you are there. ^{9}If I rise on the wings of the dawn, if I settle on the far side of the sea, ^{10}even there your hand will guide me, your right hand will hold me fast.

THANKFUL, GRATEFUL, BLESSED
February 10, 2018

Well I enjoyed a wonderful two weeks with NOTHING on my calendar. No appointments, no treatments......just NOTHING. What a blessing that was. I didn't feel my best earlier in the week - I had some headaches, wasn't sleeping great and just feeling yucky.....almost like I was trying to come down with something, but thankfully, that passed and I felt much better as the week went on. I enjoyed a lot of Netflix time.

***Side note - if you have Netflix and HAVE NOT watched Parenthood......oh my......add that to your list of MUST SEE TV. It really is an awesome show!! Yeah - I mighta watched all 6 seasons in record time! #allthefeels #missthebravermans #reallifestuff

Wednesday I had my follow-up appointment with my medical oncologist. My blood work was incredible she said. My potassium was a bit low - but other than that, everything looked fantastic. Praise God!

My radiation burns are healing nicely. The area under my arm pit is almost completely healed. We discussed immunotherapy and she put me on Tamoxifen for the next 10 years. I admit I was startled when she said 10 years - most folks I know that have taken Tamoxifen have only been on it for 5 years......but as we all know, things change.

There are new studies out indicating that taking tamoxifen for 10 years reduced the risk of breast cancer recurrence and death more than taking tamoxifen 5 years......so there ya go.

As with any drug - there's a host of potential side effects.......so the plan is for me to start on the Tamoxifen and go back to the doctor in April to see how I'm tolerating the drug. I hope and pray that I don't have any issues with it - but she assured me there were other options for me if this one didn't work out. I will go back next month for a bone-density test. So between follow ups with the surgeon, medical oncologist and radiation oncologist - my Duke My Chart is already full of return appointments set up for the rest of the year.

They said the first year is the worst - lots of follow-ups and return visits. I will see the surgeon every 6 months for 2 years. I'm already scheduled to return to the surgeon for a visit and a mammogram in May. But......the hard stuff is behind me. I can handle random appointments and tests for sure. These last 9 months have seemed like an eternity and then they seem to have passed rather quickly.

So much has happened.......I have encountered so much GOOD over the past 9 months. I have been loved on like nobody's business. From family, friends and folks I didn't even know.

I have felt the overwhelming power of prayer - and the peace that only God can give us. I've been moved to tears when I had friends say "I was up and down all night praying for you" and I've been the recipient of so much love and kindness in so many forms (cards, food, texts, visits, calls, gifts, money, transportation, prayers, etc).

I will be forever grateful.....and I know I got a little slack on thank you notes.....but please know that I appreciate every act of kindness that has been shown to me and my family during all this mess. Several folks have asked if I'll continue blogging. My initial thought is this......I pray my life is uneventful enough that I won't have much to say! :-) But......if you know me.......you know I'm typically not ever at a loss for words no matter how mundane and uneventful life may be. So we'll just see. Stay tuned!

My prayer has been that God would take my **MESS** and turn it into a **MESS**age.......and for the rest of my life, I will continue to praise Him for the many ways He has blessed me always.......but especially over the past year.....and I will continue to share my personal testimony of how He saw me through one of the toughest battles of my life.

I have been praying for God to reveal to me my "purpose"......and I trust that He will answer me......in His time.

Until next time,

Sonja

Acts 20:24 The Message (MSG)
[22-24] *"But there is another urgency before me now. I feel compelled to go to Jerusalem. I'm completely in the dark about what will happen when I get there. I do know that it won't be any picnic, for the Holy Spirit has let me know repeatedly and clearly that there are hard times and imprisonment ahead. But that matters little. What matters most to me is to finish what God started: the job the Master Jesus gave me of letting everyone I meet know all about this incredibly extravagant generosity of God.*

A FEW OF MY FAVORITE THINGS

February 21, 2018

It's been a little while since I last posted - but I am happy to report that I have been doing well and getting stronger each and every day. My energy level is improving each day.

I'm ready to feel like my old self again.

CC was diagnosed with the Flu B on Sunday, so I was immediately put on Tamiflu in an effort to keep me well.

Yesterday I had someone share with me that a friend of theirs had recently been diagnosed with colon cancer.......and she asked me what were some of my favorite things that folks did for me.

We messaged back and forth with ideas, etc and she recommended that I do a blog post featuring my favorite things.......she said "people want to help, but don't always know how."

Well here goes........and these are in no particular order.

- **Meal Train** - having friends arrange an on-line meal train was wonderful. It allowed us to pick days we did or didn't want meal deliveries. On days when I felt like crap and didn't feel like eating - at least there were meals here for CC and Hunter. It was a true blessing. https://www.mealtrain.com

- **Silk Pillowcase** - a dear friend sent me a pink silk pillowcase and after I lost my hair from chemo. Even though my hair is growing back now - I haven't been able to give up my pillowcase! https://www.amazon.com/s/ref=nb_sb_noss_1?url=search-alias%3Daps&field-keywords=pink+silk+pillowcase

- **Chemo Bag** - I bought a Scout Bag with several pockets and used that for my chemo bag. Inside I packed the following: blanket, phone charger, hand sanitizer, orange tic tacs (to help with the taste of saline when they flushed my port), snacks, lip balm, something to read, hand wipes, ACT lozenges for dry mouth, https://www.scoutbags.com/dippin-dots-pocket-rocket-pocket-tote-bag?utm_source=google&utm_medium=cpc&adpos=1o6&UTM_campaign=general&scid=scplp16150&sc_intid=16150&gclid=Cj0KCQiAzrTUBRCnARIsAL0mqcwPnVAYXPwFymRa8-Apo-ruBdzfMIqe4dS4HNLe1Jd945nrydWFu-kaAjQQEALw_wcB

- **Transportation** - having friends and family arrange to transport me to doctor's appointments, chemotherapy sessions and radiation treatments was such a blessing.

- **Journal & great pens** - having a journal to record visits, calls, thoughts, etc. was very therapeutic.

- **Gift cards** - during chemo when I was battling with mouth sores, soups were about the only thing I could eat. We have a deli in town that has a variety of soups. I was gifted several rounds of gift cards there and they were such a blessing. But gift cards in general are great - that would allow the family the ability to grab dinner on the go at times.

- **Books** - hands down this was my favorite read. https://www.amazon.com/Fight-Back-Joy-Celebrate-Greatest/dp/1617950890

- **Milkshakes** - on days when eating just wasn't in the cards......and nothing sounded good - a banana milk shake was my go-to. I had folks call or text at random times to say "I'm in town, can I bring you a milkshake?" YESSSSS please!

- **Adult Coloring Books & Pencils** - these offer a great escape when you're sitting and waiting in the hospital.

- **Cute Caps** - these are definitely a MUST - even if they lose their hair in the summer time, your head still gets cold. Do you knit or crochet? Even better! Make them some super cute caps!

- **Lip balm** - chemo really really dried out my lips - so I kept lip balm on my nightstand, in the car, on the end table, in my coat pocket........you get the picture.

- **Cleaning** - whether you go and do a few loads of laundry or clean out the refrigerator - those are truly great gifts. Or maybe you prefer to pay a cleaning service to come in and clean - that works too!

- **Port shirt** - these are fantastic for chemo. The zippers allow for super easy access to the port. They come in several different colors and long and short sleeves! http://www.survivorroom.com/chemo-port-accessible-womens-pink-long-sleeve-shirt-by-comfy-chemo/?utm_medium=googleshopping&utm_source=bc

- **Cards of Encouragement** - I have received an enormous amount of cards since my diagnosis. Some days I got a bunch and then some days just a few - but I treasured each one. If you are a card sender - DO NOT underestimate the value of sending cards. They are truly treasured!

- **Goody baskets** - Gosh, I got my very first taste of Shari's Berries last summer. Can you say DELICIOUS??? Goodness these things were awesome. https://www.berries.com I also received a wonderful gift basket with lots of yummy goodness from NC. NC Country ham, pancake mix, grits, and homemade preserves. Yummy! These were gifts the entire family was able to enjoy!

- **Schedule some time to just hang out** - we really get sick of ONLY talking about cancer......I promise. I remember one day a friend came by and had lunch with me and was sharing about a work issue. She apologized for venting to me saying something like "you have cancer and here I am going on about this small issue." NO!!! I WELCOMED the distraction. Cancer patients are still normal human beings. We want to talk about kids, school, church, what's going on in the world around us, vacation plans, etc. Just schedule an hour or so to just come by, hang out and catch up. Normal feels good.

- **Therapy lunches or getaways** - I tried as much as possible to still have our weekly therapy lunches with my girls. It didn't always happen - but when I felt like it, we always tried to work something out. Again - keep doing what you've always done. And if the patient is well enough to sneak away for a few days - a girl or guys' weekend away can do wonders.

- **Shop for a wig** - losing my hair wasn't such a big deal for me - but the idea of shopping for a wig was a little scary. I was fortunate to have a wonderful friend from church who offered to take me to Raleigh to the Gallery of Wigs. A trip I truly dreaded turned into SO - MUCH - FUN! If you're a great encourager - offer to take them shopping for wigs! https://www.galleryofwigs.com

- **Make life normal for the kids** - this one was HUGE for me. My son was 14 when I was diagnosed with cancer. Fourteen is difficult enough on a good day - but factor in a mom battling cancer, and that just gets even more complicated. Having folks offer to take my child places, do things with him, invite him to movies, games, etc. -

anything to get him AWAY from the house and the constant reminder of cancer. That was a HUGE blessing to me. So if you can borrow the kid for a play date, a day at the lake, a trip to get ice cream, movies, dinner out - ANYTHING.......I promise you if you are keeping their kids engaged, that's blessing the patient also!

I'm sure I will think of many more ideas - but these were just the ones that stood out. I can promise you that no act of kindness - no matter how small or great - will go unnoticed.

I was and continue to be thankful for everything that has been done for my family and me. My "tribe" and my community showed up in big and small ways - and I am forever grateful! I hope this list helps those of you who were looking for ideas.

And by all means - if any of you have great ideas you'd like to add, please send me a note and I'll add your favorites also!

Blessings,

Sonja

Luke 6:38 New International Version (NIV)
[38] *Give, and it will be given to you. A good measure, pressed down, shaken together and running over, will be poured into your lap. For with the measure you use, it will be measured to you.*

Hebrews 13:2 New International Version (NIV)
[2] *Do not forget to show hospitality to strangers, for by so doing some people have shown hospitality to angels without knowing it.*

THINKING OUT LOUD
March 7, 2018

Well it's been a minute since I've posted. Things got a little crazy around here. CC was diagnosed with the flu in mid-February.......and my doctor put me on Tamiflu the same day he was diagnosed and I tried as hard as I could to stay away from his cooties. I slept in the spare bedroom, disinfected the house like a villain, diffused essential oils, washed, washed, washed my hands, drank elderberry syrup.......you name it, I did my best to avoid it. What's that they say about the best laid plans? Well - the flu caught me too!

Crazy enough we had both had the flu shot this year (this was the very first year I've EVER had it, but my oncologists strongly recommended that I take it). CC was diagnosed on a Sunday and by the following Friday - I was feeling like crap! The worst part was the terrible cough and congestion.

Because of the timing of my illness, there was some concern that I may have pneumonitis (often a side effect of radiation that can show up a month or more after treatment). My radiation oncologist ordered x-rays to be sure what we were dealing with.

Thank goodness there was no pneumonitis - but she called me later that day to say that I, too, had tested positive for Flu B. Are you kidding me?

I'm happy to report that we are both feeling much better at this time. Praise God! That was a rough few weeks.

I still have a terrible nagging cough - but who knows if that's from the flu or from this crazy weather that now has everything blooming outside! My strength is coming back day by day. I'm finding it easier to be out and about doing things for longer periods of time.

Slowly but surely life is getting back to normal. Tomorrow I have an appointment for a bone density test - they ordered that after they put me on the Tamoxifen. Guess we need a baseline reading on my bone health. Hopefully that will be a quick trip tomorrow. I have enjoyed not having to travel to Duke on a daily basis these past few weeks!

I seem to be adjusting okay to the Tamoxifen. Yeah - I started experiencing major "power surges" literally within the first 24 hours of starting the meds. They occur sporadically all through the day and night. Fun times!

I haven't felt like I've experienced any "mood swings" - which seems to be a common side effect of the meds. My guys haven't seemed to complain, so I hope we can avoid that one! I'm finding that nothing really sounds good when it comes to food. Food tastes pretty normal now so that's a good thing......but even foods I have always loved just don't appeal to me like before. Or I'll spend all day thinking about the yummy dinner I'm gonna cook and then by the time it's ready - it's not appealing to me at all. I dunno.

Maybe this is a good thing? Maybe I'll lose some weight? Fat chance!

My hair is coming back and it's grown a bunch over the past few weeks. Many folks have asked me if my hair is coming back in its natural color.

HELLO PEOPLE.......I'd been coloring my hair for so long, who the heck remembers what my natural color looked like??? Last I knew, it was almost black. Now it's coming back baby soft and very much in a salt and pepper color! I haven't noticed ANY. SINGLE. BIT. OF. CURL.........DANGIT! I had sooooo hoped I'd have some ringlets! Or at the very least a little bit of body! I'm still holding out for that! I want Melba Thompson hair! :-)

Here's wishing each of you a wonderful rest of the week. I challenge each of you to find some JOY in each day. Even in the midst of chaos - look for the blessing that is tucked away somewhere around the corner. Choose to be optimistic rather than pessimistic.......choose to see the glass as half full rather than half empty......and by golly, be nice to yourself every now and then. Right Tina Morris?

It's okay to buy yourself a bouquet of flowers or treat yourself to something special.

But ya'll......seriously......with all the crap that's going on in the world around us......there's a lot of bad stuff, but a heckuva lot of good stuff too......and we may not be able to do much but one thing we can all do is just BE KIND. It's just that easy. Need some ideas?

https://www.lifehack.org/articles/communication/30-ways-kind-and-happier.html

Choose kindness........every time. Bessings!

Sonja

Colossians 3:12-14 The Message (MSG)
12-14So, chosen by God for this new life of love, dress in the wardrobe God picked out for you: compassion, kindness, humility, quiet strength, discipline. Be even-tempered, content with second place, quick to forgive an offense. Forgive as quickly and completely as the Master forgave you. And regardless of what else you put on, wear love. It's your basic, all-purpose garment. Never be without it.

PNEU-MO-WHAT?
March 14, 2018

If you remember, on my last update, I was sad to report that I had been diagnosed with Flu B. Thankfully - I had just finished a round of Tamiflu, so I think I was able to kick the flu a little quicker because of that. About a week after my diagnosis, I was feeling better thank the Lord.

Last Thursday I was scheduled for my baseline Bone Density Test. That was one of the fastest appointments I've had at Duke. I was called back before my appointment time, changed into a gown and less than 5 minutes later, I was dressed and on my way back home. What a pleasant surprise.

My radiation oncologist had made a return visit for me last Friday to follow up from the flu. She had said if I was better, I could cancel it......and I seriously thought about it.....especially since I had just been to Duke on Thursday - who wanted to go back again if it wasn't NECESSARY. The only thing holding me back was the fact that I still had a very nasty cough that just wouldn't seem to go away. But I'd talked to several folks who were recovering from the flu and most of them said the cough just hung around forever - so I kinda thought it was just part of the process.

Of course, I mentioned to my mom that I was considering NOT going to the doctor and she quickly informed me that she thought I should definitely go and see what they said about my cough. Hopefully it was nothing - but better safe than sorry. And truthfully - she was right. She even went with me to the appointment. (I think mostly so she could make sure I went and didn't take off shopping!)

My lungs sounded great when the PA checked me out. She agreed, however, that my cough was going on a bit long and she felt like it was prudent that we investigate it a little further. She ordered a CT scan and I was blessed to be able to have one that day within an hour. Some days you just hit the hospital lottery! I walked over to the Medical Pavilion to have my CT scan and was called back before I could get seated good. The CT took about 3.5 minutes and then I was on my way.

I wasn't really expecting to know anything from the CT scan til probably the following week.....but I actually received a voicemail from the PA Friday night about 7:41 saying she was just calling me to follow up on the CT and if I hadn't heard back from her by Monday morning, to give her a call on Monday.......which I did. When we were finally able to connect on Monday evening - she informed me that the good news was there was **no signs of cancer** ....HUGE sigh of relief.......but that there was evidence of pneumonitis. Grrrrr.

My doctor had told me of the *possibility* of pneumonitis literally the very first day I consulted with her....but of course we had hoped that we wouldn't have to deal with it.

For those of you who are like me and may had never heard of pneumonitis before -

> **Pneumonitis (noo-moe-NIE-tis)** is a general term that refers to inflammation of lung tissue. Technically, pneumonia is a type of pneumonitis because the infection causes inflammation. Pneumonitis, however, is usually used by doctors to refer to noninfectious causes of lung inflammation. If pneumonitis is

undetected or left untreated, you may gradually develop chronic pneumonitis, which can result in scarring (fibrosis) in the lungs.

(Above definition from www.mayoclinic.org/diseases-conditions/pneumonitis/symptoms-causes/syc-20352623)

Pneumonitis, a noninfectious inflammation of the lungs, is a side effect associated with several cancer treatments, including radiation and chemotherapy as well as newer targeted drugs and immunotherapies. The symptoms range from mild to severe respiratory symptoms but may not appear until weeks to months into treatment — and sometimes long after treatments end — leading to frequent misdiagnoses, particularly because the symptoms resemble those of pneumonia. (Definition from www.curetoday.com/publications/cure/2015/ summer-2015/pneumonitis-a-delayed-reaction)

If you'd like to read more - here's a link with some additional information: www.curetoday.com/publications/cure/2015/ summer-2015/pneumonitis-a-delayed-reaction

According to the doctor - one of the types of chemo that I received can cause pneumonitis as well as the radiation......so I kinda had a double whammy. On top of that, the breathing issues I experienced when I had those few Taxol treatments already had my system compromised a bit. Even though the doctor had mentioned this all along - of course we had HOPED and PRAYED that I would avoid it. But that wasn't to be the case. Soooo...... they put me on a high dose of steroids for the next 5 weeks and I pray that will take care of. They have all ready warned me if I'm not better at the 5 week mark, that we may do an additional 3 weeks of steroids. Whatever it takes. The Good Lord has seen me through the past 11 months.....I have faith He will see me through this hurdle too. (Gosh is it possible that next month will be a year since all this started???)

That being said.......to quote Uncle Joe from Madea, I may be "big as a Buick" by the time I finish these steroids. So if you are looking for me any time in the next 5 weeks, if I'm not at home, check the closest buffets! :-) So.......as bad as I hate to say it.......Mom was right. It was prudent for me to take the time to go back to the doctor to have my cough investigated. While we didn't get the news we had hoped - at least we know and have a plan. I'm glad I went and let them check me out a little further. Better safe than sorry.

Now you know that when you see me and I'm still coughing like a villain, I'm NOT contagious......but just having a difficult time shedding this cough. Hopefully I will start to see some improvement soon.

On a brighter note......today we celebrated Hunter's 15th birthday. How is it possible that my child now has his learner's permit? God blessed us with a wonderful son. He's kind, sweet, sensitive, caring, smart, compassionate and just an all-around good kid. I am so proud to be his mom!

Prayers for a great rest of your week.

Sonja

Romans 15:13 New International Version (NIV)
[13] May the God of hope fill you with all joy and peace as you trust in him, so that you may overflow with hope by the power of the Holy Spirit.

HAPPY SPRING, Y'ALL!
March 20, 2018

I'm happy to report that today I checked off the first week of steroids for the pneumonitis (one week down, hopefully only 4 more to go)! I've felt good all things considered - the worst part has just been the cough that just doesn't seem to want to go away. I know.......it just takes time. The cough seems to be more annoying first thing in the morning and then again late at night. Thankfully, I'm able to sleep now without having to take any cough medicine......so that's a step in the right direction. This, too, shall pass!

I was at a meeting at church last night and of course, was coughing off and on. I know the first thing folks think when I start barking is "oh gosh, she's contagious." Fortunately - I can't give you pneumonitis. But I totally get folks wanting to keep their distance!

I find myself celebrating the weeks when I don't have to go to Duke for any doctor visits. It's funny how sometimes even the smallest of victories are worth claiming! I do have to return to Durham tomorrow for an appointment - but this time it's with the endodontist to complete the second and hopefully last part of my root canal. Praying the second part is as painless as the first. If you are ever in need of a great endodontist, check out Dr. Deborah Conner in Durham, NC. They have an awesome staff there!

So I've been asked over the past few weeks about updates to my recovery and I've enjoyed sharing my success/progress by this crazy yard stick:

BBC (Before Breast Cancer) - my friends made fun of me for going to the grocery store MULTIPLE times a week. I know.....kinda crazy but over the years I've tried meal planning for a week and it almost always ended up in wasted food. CC may call at 3:00 pm and say "I just had lunch, don't worry about dinner" - or "I'm working late, you just get something for you and Hunter"........or we might get an invitation to meet friends for dinner or in the best cases - be invited by family for a real old fashioned home-cooked meal......and this crew REFUSES to turn down that kind of food. Anyway - weekly planning just doesn't work for us - so the result of that is that I was typically at the grocery store 3-4 times a week.

Last week, as I stood in line at Food Lion waiting to check out - a friend was in line ahead of me. She turned around and asked me how I was doing.......and in that instant.......it suddenly hit me. I couldn't help but stand there and chuckle to myself. This was the second day in a row that I was at Food Lion getting items for dinner and that hadn't happened in a very long time! I laughed and told my friend that it appeared I was back to normal......given that I was finding myself back in my old habit of grocery shopping several times a week! It was crazy and cool all at the same time. As crazy as my grocery shopping habit is - it was pretty awesome to stand there and realize that - WOW - maybe my life is getting back to normal! So.....right there.......in the check out line at Food Lion - I felt like God was patting me on the back and saying "we are almost there, my friend."

My energy level is increasing daily. I find that my stamina is also increasing. I still have a bit of a "sinking spell" each afternoon typically between 3-5pm - but I just try to stop and catch my breath......and take a power nap if need be.

Baby steps. I'll take them!

I feel like a spring flower.......pushing through the dirt.......a little bit at a time.......but eventually, all that pushing pays off and a beautiful flower emerges. Bring on the spring!

My heart is heavy tonight as I learned that a dear friend and fellow cancer warrior, Roger, went to be the with Lord today. He put up an amazing fight over the past three years. He and his wife were extra special to me......and I am truly a better person because I knew them. Roger definitely showed me how to fight with grace and dignity. While I will miss his big hugs when I walk into church on Sundays.......I celebrate that He has met our Lord and Savior and his suffering is no more. My thoughts and prayers go out to his wife and children.

Last night at a meeting at church, my friend Lisa shared a wonderful devotion. It really spoke to me. It talked about a man who looked in the mirror every day and asked himself "what are you going to do for Jesus today?"

What a powerful message in just eight small words! It really got my attention. What are YOU going to do for Jesus today? How awesome would it be if we all woke up each day with a desire to do even just ONE thing for Jesus each day. I challenge you to give it a shot. It doesn't have to be HUGE......maybe it's buying a meal for someone, or calling a shut-in, or sending a card of encouragement to a young teen, or running an errand for an elderly neighbor, paying for the person's coffee in line behind you at the coffee shop, text a Bible verse to a friend who may be struggling.

There are countless ways we can do something for Jesus and share His love with others. I'd LOVE to hear ideas you have of other awesome and creative things we could do for Jesus.

Wishing you a very blessed week.

Hugs!

Sonja

Song of Songs 2:11-12 New International Version (NIV)
[11]See! The winter is past; the rains are over and gone. [12]Flowers appear on the earth; the season of singing has come, the cooing of doves is heard in our land.

HE IS RISEN!
April 5, 2018

Well it's been a good little spell since I updated my blog. As I sat here and realized just how long it's been - I had to smile and say "thanks God" because the truth of the matter is, I've been feeling great and been quite busy going about life. How awesome is it that I've been so busy I completely didn't think about blogging! Small steps!

These steroids must be working........I'm feeling much better and no coughing, etc., even though I still have another week of meds left before I complete the regimen. I will be thankful to finish up the steroids. Good grief ya'll.......I'm eating every thing in sight! I'm not a huge "sweets" person - I typically prefer two helpings of meat and potatoes over sweets.......but lately.......oh my! We have been making s'mores in the oven wayyyy more than we should........and I made a lemon pie because I could not stop thinking about lemon pie! Totally out of character for me! I will be big as a Buick if I don't hurry up and get off these steroids! Lordy!

So we spent Easter with our family at Myrtle Beach. We had a great time - laughing, eating, shopping and just hanging out. For several years now the Methodist church a few blocks away has held Easter Sunrise Service on the beach a couple blocks up from our condo. We were there the very first year they held the service and it was a handful of folks in attendance and lots of technical difficulties.....you know, the typical growing pains when you are trying something new. The next year there were a few more people.......and golly gee, I'd be afraid to guess how many folks showed up this past Sunday for the Sunrise Service. HUNDREDS for sure! It was an enormous crowd. Kudos to the folks at Trinity UMC for all their hard work in organizing this wonderful worship service

Easter has always been a special time of year for me........but now it holds even more significance to me personally. You see, last year Easter came a little later in the year. It was on April 15th to be exact.

But last year, CC wasn't able to go with us to the beach for Easter because he had to work. I am too old for all this "selfie" craze (thank goodness)! So we were sitting out on the beach, and I took a "selfie" and texted it to him to say thanks for working hard so I could play hard (or something to that effect).

I had forgotten about that picture until recently when I was going through the photos on my phone. I saw my picture and took note of the date. April 15th, 2017. Unbelievable!

This picture was taken 3 days before my yearly physical with Dr. Frenduto when this whole mess started.

Three days before my personal "shit storm!" How crazy that I could look so "well" and "healthy" in that picture and not have any idea what was lurking in my body.

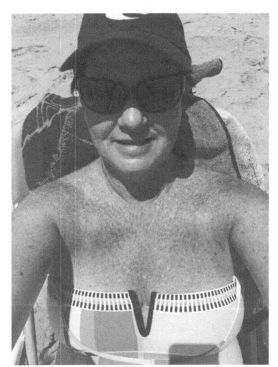

Looks can be deceiving. Little did this gal know what was lurking around the corner!

2017 was full of doctors' appointments, tests, chemo and radiation, and unfortunately my treatments spilled over into 2018 as well....but we finally wrapped that mess up. And this Easter.......I was back at the beach with my family.........fully aware of just how blessed I was to be there......things had come full-circle and I'd celebrated my own personal "resurrection" experience, so to speak. I'd endured some dark days over the past year - but God saw me through those tough days and continues to guide me through the days ahead. To think that Jesus endured the Cross for me......for my sins......for my cancer!!

So this Easter was pretty stinking special. As I watched the sun rise on Easter Sunday.........I was pure thankful. I find myself living more "in the moment" now. Truly trying to soak every thing in.......and not miss a thing.

I know it's a little late given Easter has passed - but the video below is a favorite of mine. No matter how dark your Friday(s)........it's okay, because Sunday's coming! It's worth sharing even if it's a little late!

https://www.youtube.com/watch?v=cikenKl92Og

I'd like to give a big shout out to my friend and fellow cancer warrior Miriam. She finished up her treatments today. Well done, my friend! So happy you have this behind you now! God is good. She rocked this cancer #likeaboss!

Happy Weekend! Make every minute of it count!

Sonja

Matthew 28:6 The Message (MSG)
5-6 The angel spoke to the women: "There is nothing to fear here. I know you're looking for Jesus, the One they nailed to the cross. He is not here. He was raised, just as he said. Come and look at the place where he was placed. 7 "Now, get on your way quickly and tell his disciples, 'He is risen from the dead. He is going on ahead of you to Galilee. You will see him there.' That's the message."

Made in the USA
Columbia, SC
01 February 2019